Fitness for Beginners

How to Assess Your Fitness Level and Create a Personal Exercise Plan

(Get in Shape and Stay in Shape for the Rest of Your Life Without Going to the Gym)

Daniel Lane

Published By **Bella Frost**

Daniel Lane

Fitness for Beginners: How to Assess Your Fitness Level and Create a Personal Exercise Plan (Get in Shape and Stay in Shape for the Rest of Your Life Without Going to the Gym)

ISBN   978-1-998927-06-7

No part of this guidebook shall be reproduced in any form without permission in writing from the publisher except in the case of brief quotations embodied in critical articles or reviews.

Legal & Disclaimer

The information contained in this book is not designed to replace or take the place of any form of medicine or professional medical advice. The information in this book has been provided for educational & entertainment purposes only.

The information contained in this book has been compiled from sources deemed reliable, and it is accurate to the best of the Author's knowledge; however, the Author cannot guarantee its accuracy and validity and cannot be held liable for any errors or omissions. Changes are periodically made to this book. You must consult your doctor or get professional medical advice before using any of the suggested remedies, techniques, or information in this book.

Table Of Contents

Chapter 1: THE CORE STRENGTHENING

A flat stomach and 6 p.C. Abs have been a regular hassle rely of dialogue in the fitness global. No surprise, for it does signify fitness, vigor and problem. A individual who has a flat stomach and six p.C. Abs have emerge as not able to do it in a single day. He or she set apart time, strength and assets every day a terrific manner to accumulate this aim. Expect to do the equal, for it's miles your strength of mind with a view to permit you to be successful.

Attaining a extraordinary set of abs does want some of willpower and everyone may have it via way of doing to matters on the equal time, and people are body fat bargain and center strengthening.

Keep in thoughts that each of those artwork hand in hand. For instance, you can do some of middle strengthening carrying sports but in case your abs are included via a layer of greater fat, your six percentage abs will stay invisible. Likewise, in case you circulate on an intensive weight-reduction plan to lose all of that fat, your abs received't form into the incredible six % that best a exercising can shape it to.

Body Fat Reduction

Men have to intention for approximately a 10 percent body fat until their abs must start to show, while ladies need to goal for approximately sixteen percentage. To recognize how hundreds your cutting-edge-day frame fats percent is, you can have it measured via doing the skinfold caliper method or the bioelectrical impedance approach. Health experts is probably able to administer those assessments. You can also check on-line for body fat calculators that may provide you with rougher estimate in case you degree sure additives of your body with a measuring tape.

The most effective way to explain the method of body fats cut price is this: eat a brilliant deal plenty less, and burn extra. Food is made of energy or electricity, and in case you are not able to expend the quantity of power which you have ate up the body will keep it within the form of fats deposits. You will observe the most crucial healthy eating plan guidelines to help you get a flat belly.

Core Strengthening

Specific sports activities can purpose the strengthening of your center, in any other case called your "powerhouse." This is your belly location, and it serves to keep collectively your better and reduce frame additives in addition to maintaining your internal organs in area. The six percentage abs are composed of muscle corporations called the rectus abdominis however it ought to no longer be the handiest aim muscle to artwork on. You can even want to increase your lateral belly muscle businesses called the transversus abdominis and your inner and outside belly obliques to get a leaner waist. Note that even as you inhale and keep your stomach in, you're clearly contracting your transversus abdominis.

You becomes familiar with the first-rate sporting occasions that intention to boom your six p.C. Abs. It is quite recommended which you memorize those actions so you can efficiently exercise them at some point of your software program.

Developing a Strong Core Is a Must

Let's speak physics for a few seconds now, we should? Don't fear, I'm no longer going to head all Friedmann on you and begin losing horrifying equations that'll provide you with nightmares for days. I certainly want to talk approximately breaking factors.

Answer me this: typically, in which is any item at its weakest? When you bend a piece of timber and keep to increase the stress little by little, what happens?

Any frame is nearly constantly at its weakest at the center... and the human body is not any exception! If it's frail at the middle, it'll smash like a twig at the same time as positioned underneath stress. As the pronouncing goes, a sequence is high-quality as sturdy as its weakest link. The center is the hinge of the body; it requires greater care and hobby to ensure it keeps the entire chain strong, solid and wholesome.

Working the middle is an absolute prerequisite to reaching any of the greater advanced frame weight movements... However you don't need to be worried with calisthenics to gain the rewards of unique abs schooling.

In fact, strengthening the abdominals has been confirmed to boom your ordinary universal performance in any region, some aspect your pastimes or profession. It should make you quicker or have you ever hit (together collectively along with your fist or your foot) a excellent deal harder.

How? Well, to move lower back to the frame-chain photo we referred to, your center is the principle link connecting the 2 extremities of your body which are your legs and your trunk. When you accomplish any undertaking, from kicking a soccer to sporting a heavy bag, your abs will constantly get solicited at one factor or each extraordinary. Either at once, whilst the movement originates from your center, or in a roundabout manner because the pressure you've generated on your legs travels through your center to reach your fingers (or vice versa.) Like while you're throwing a fastball.

At the very least, your middle will play a stabilizing role and avoid power leakage. In quick, your abs are the concept and guide from which any motion earnings momentum. Keep them in negative state of affairs and undergo the effects!

If that wasn't cause sufficient to be able to start a center strengthening software program program, recall the ones unique advantages:

• Working your center will offer you with advanced stability: via assisting to stabilize your torso and limbs, stronger abs will growth your stability and moreover make you flow into and change recommendations plenty quicker (extraordinary for soccer gamers and one of a kind athletes who need to trap their warring parties off balance);

• Working your center will decorate your breathing: precise center schooling will even pork up your diaphragm that is essential to the respiration procedure. It will make every simply taken into consideration one among your inspirations a bargain greater deeper and effective. Thanks to a better oxygenation of your muscle businesses and your thoughts, you will enjoy lots a great deal much less stressed and more alert;

• Working your center will improve your digestion: feeling a piece bloated or constipated lately? Train the abs! With the wearing events we'll see underneath, you may no longer handiest decorate up but enlarge your abdominals which, in the occasion that they're too quick or stiff, can squeeze your inner organs and prevent right meals assimilation;

• Working your center will beautify your posture: pretty self-explanatory. Since your abs assist stabilize your over again, improving their electricity and flexibility will pass an prolonged way in the direction of obtaining the proper posture;

• Working your middle will save you lower back pain and restriction injuries: a corollary to the preceding element, better abs can even advocate less chance of developing over again pain as you'll be recognition straighter and your spine gets more help. For the same motive, you'll gain from greater protection in opposition to any wonder, torsion or pressure you could hold and that could bring about an harm;

• Working your middle will make your bones a awesome deal more potent: very last but now not least, just like with body weight education, via targeted to your abs and setting your bones under stress, you may lead them to stronger through the years because the introduced stress of the physical video video games will in flip growth their density.

As you may see, quite some sweet advantages all and sundry seeking to carry out at his extraordinary can be stupid not to take advantage of!

But it's less difficult stated than achieved, right? Can you simply lie down, do a couple take a seat down-ups, and anticipate to appear like Gerard Butler within the 300's at the same time as you rise up? You need!

What's for splendid is that with all of the crap we pay attention or take a look at about in magazines, not to mention the ones late-night time time infomercials that never seem to expire of "miracle" merchandise that sell for a pinnacle rate and that promise to get you ripped at the same time as you sleep, it is able to get near no longer viable for the amateur to type between truth and BS. To understand precisely what to do and avoid like the plague.

You will find out the way you could also flip this susceptible thing of yours into truly considered one in all your number one strengths. So, in case you're prepared, buckle up and allow's claim that superhero six-percentage you've been searching ahead to!

Chapter 2: BENEFITS OF HAVING STRONG ABDOMINAL MUSCLES

Having robust abs is critical for not excellent athletes, but furthermore non-athletes. Located at the middle of your body, stomach muscle tissues play a important role in stability, stability, and normal physical power. Not most effective this, reinforced stomach muscle tissues help your once more and assist in preserving right posture. When your abs are sculpted and in shape, they appearance attractive and assist with physical activities. Ripped abs do more than sincerely turn heads. With more potent abs, you experience an advanced health diploma, and as a end end result are capable of with out issue perform everyday obligations in addition to better conventional usual overall performance in sports activities.

Metabolism Boost

According to Mayo Clinic, people with extra muscle burn extra energy and feature a higher metabolism. The more potent your abs are, the more power are burnt so you can hold them. With higher metabolism, you're in more manage of your weight. Compared to fat tissue, the style of power burned on a each day foundation is greater in the case of muscle tissues. This way the bigger and stronger the abs, the better the metabolism fee this is proper away correlated for your primary fitness.

Better Posture

Having a ripped body does not simplest ought to do with appearance, but it additionally allows maintain your spine in an upright function. What's greater, an upright posture will beautify your appearance and make you appearance taller and on top of things. Strengthening your abs allows pull on your stomach and stand up straight.

Lower Risk of Back Injuries

Getting an brilliant set of abs not fine gives on your frame aesthetics, however also lowers the chance of lower again damage. Primarily the cause for decrease over again ache is susceptible stomach muscle mass and bulging weight around your belly. When you burn stomach fat and tighten your abs, this takes pressure off your again and reduces your risk of lower back injuries.

Less Pressure on Joints

The stronger the abs, the more stable your frame is, which means that that less stress on joints. Since the muscle groups surrounds the joints, the superb way to protect it's far to reinforce the muscle mass. Improving your middle strength will help reduce the hazard of harm if you are actively participating in sports.

A Longer Life

With an notable tummy, you may experience an prolonged lifestyles expectancy. According to a Canadian check conducted for over 13 years, people with the weakest abs had greater than double the dying charge in assessment to people with the strongest midsections.

Increased Sports Efficiency

Core is a buzz phrase within the worldwide of sports sports. Strong center allows enhance everyday typical performance in each game, be it on foot, gymnastics, soccer, swimming, basketball, cricket, and biking.

Techniques for Building Strong Abs

The stronger the abs, the healthier the spine, the better your posture may be. With more potent abs and a greater wholesome spine, you may effectively transfer energy from your decrease body to the palms, making actions a good deal much less complicated.

Your middle is based at the muscle groups for manual, no longer like one-of-a-kind frame components that rely on bones. You cannot lose stomach fat thru simply doing extra ab carrying activities. Training the entire frame with immoderate intensity workout workouts will help to burn that greater fat.

Crunching, rotating, or churning won't be the right technique to get better abs. A University of South Florida studies record suggests, it's the free-weight physical sports activities that spark off the center muscle businesses that will help you get the desired abs. As in competition to commonplace notion, muscle-specific, floor-based truly sports, along side sit down down-ups, do now not prompt center muscle groups.

Merely training the sporting sports activities will now not help a good deal; alternatively, it's miles the coordination among all muscle groups that allows construct strength. In order to have a ripped body, you need to first bring your belly fat diploma down, due to the fact your six percent abs are hidden below that layer of fats.

Shift your recognition to cardiovascular education, resistance schooling, purpose setting, healthful way of life alternatives, rest and restoration.

One of the biggest errors people make whilst seeking to accelerate fats loss is with the useful resource of education the wrong sort of aerobic exercise. Most people take delivery of as genuine with that prolonged, low intensity aerobic workout workouts assist boost up fats loss, which is inaccurate. High depth c program languageperiod cardio training allows burn a notable amount of fat, and need to be targeted straight away to collect six percentage abs.

Why Your Abs Are Not Showing

If you have got got have been given been making everyday trips to the gym and running out hard but however now not seeing chiseled abs, you're in truth making a mistake somewhere.

• Too Much Fat Around the Abdominal Wall

If there is an excessive amount of subcutaneous fats around your abs area, your six percent abs obtained't be visible as they will be hiding beneath. The fat will not leave with out problems except you workout hard and eat right. So step one you may want to take in the direction of getting a ripped body is to clean up your food regimen and take a look at a smart meal plan.

Doing so will assist decrease the overall fats percentage to your body and find your abs. Without clever meal making plans, your workout exercises in the gym will not be almost as powerful.

• Doing simplest crunches

Training your muscular tissues simplest to flex through crunches will not assist prompt each muscle. In order to get a toned frame, with muscle tissue that pop, the abdominals need to examine from specific dimensions and angles. Try a combination of sports activities, in preference to training without a doubt one kind. Deadlifts, planks, and useless insects are maximum of the severa carrying sports that allow you to gain your goal of six percentage abs.

17

• Try to crunch away belly fat

It is a incorrect notion that with crunches, you may shed stomach fat. Rather, you can't lose fat particularly regions through education a selected frame issue difficult. You cannot lose your intestine via appearing abdominal carrying activities, since you can't control wherein the fats burns for your frame. Instead, attempt to burn your frame fats through a mixture of food plan, aerobic, and resistance schooling.

Consistency is the important element almost about firming your body. Religiously following a healthful consuming and exercise everyday will allow your abs to come to be defined for decades to come back back.

Nutritional and Diet Advice for Six Pack Abs

There isn't a few element like a brief fats loss solution. But if you eat proper and educate tough, you can get a decent tummy, with properly-described six percentage abs.

• Go green

Green greens are not most effective properly for substantial health, however additionally for your abs. As rich belongings of vitamins, nutrients, dietary fiber, and calcium and espresso in caloric consumption, green leafy vegetables ought to be a essential part of your healthy weight loss program so that you can sculpt amazing abs.

The exquisite takeaway from greens is that you can not pass incorrect with vegetables. Load your food with veggies, and refill with terrific vitamins. Not handiest this, you'll lose the temptation to make dangerous nutritional selections.

• Say no to processed sugar

Processed sugar is the maximum important foe at the same time as you are attempting to get chiseled abs. If you consume a further of processed sugars, opportunities are it's far going to be stored as fats within the frame if you fail to metabolize it fast. A sugar-wealthy weight-reduction plan will conflict together with your quest to getting a toned body.

Fruits do no longer fall under this class, as they haven't been stripped in their natural fiber. Since they aren't processed, they metabolize slowly, now not like processed sugars.

• Drink more water

Water is the outstanding beverage for a healthful and ripped frame. So whether or not or not you are seeking out fitness or abs, make it a aspect to drink masses of water in some unspecified time in the future of the day, in region of gulping sugary beverages and soda liquids. Water improves metabolism and aids in digestion, which means which you get leaner faster. Not fantastic this, water intake eliminates pollution from body, consequently decreasing aches and assisting to enhance the advent of abs.

• Eat cautiously

Eating sparsely does no longer advise ravenous yourself. It satisfactory technique eating simplest the favored quantity of food which you need to satisfy your hunger. Subjecting yourself to starvation and deprivation is incorrect. Food is meant to be enjoyed, and you could do so in case you want to live healthful, healthy and characteristic an terrific set of abs.

• Have wonderful proteins & important carbs

Protein want to be an critical a part of your nutritional routine in case you need to get a lean, described appearance, because it fuels the muscle tissue and permits of their rebuilding after a tough exercise. In fact, your every day protein intake need to be 0.Eight - 2 grams in line with kg of your weight. Like proteins, your frame goals remarkable carbs. Include greater end result to your meals and reduce back on sugary and processed foods. Doing so will assist strip away that bulging belly faster and rapid attain your six % ab purpose! Additionally, you want some amount of fats to increase extraordinary abs. Nuts, avocado, and olive oil are correct resources of healthful fats.

Supplements for Building Six Pack Abs

To get a superb tummy, you need to remove greater belly fat. There are some brilliant dietary dietary supplements that you would probable want to use to shed greater fats and description your center.

L-Glutamine

As an essential amino acid, glutamine permits your frame burn fat and preserve carbs as muscle glycogen. It plays a characteristic in muscle restoration and promotes lean muscle retention, besides supporting display your hidden six percentage.

Green Tea Extract

Polyphenols in green tea are critical for each bodybuilder eyeing at that six p.C. Figure. Taking inexperienced tea extract moreover helps boost up fats burning with the beneficial resource of stimulating metabolism and assisting burn more electricity.

BCAAs

BCAAs are branched-chain amino acids that fuel muscular tissues without delay. These pass the liver, which prevents muscle breakdown, triggering protein synthesis certainly so the fats is burned and used for strength.

Caffeine

When taken before sporting activities, caffeine can boost up metabolism and help metabolize fat, because of this speeding up fat loss. Not simplest this, it gives your frame an power increase, so you can train more tough to acquire your goal.

Whey and Casein

Whey is quick digested by way of the use of manner of the body. Additionally, its capability to raise glutathione, which improves immune function and reduces oxidative stress in athletes, which otherwise contributes to muscle fatigue. By supplementing your weight-reduction plan with whey protein will will let you train greater hard and longer.

Casein is a high-quality addition in your diet plan while you are considering fat loss and looking to get a ripped body. Since it's far digested slowly, Casein protein powder is superb used while you are searching out a slow-release protein on your muscular tissues.

Chapter 3: HOW TO MEASURE YOUR BODY FAT PERCENTAGE

The number one preference, simply, desires to be the DXA (for Dual Energy X-Ray Absorptiometry.) Sounds like a today's thriller weapon in development through DARPA, right? By making use of densitometry, this approach permits a particular calculation of your bones, muscle groups and fat %, to at the least one decimal region.

Here's how we're going to get our percentage then, right?

We'll additionally ought to overlook about using the BMI, as is often advocated through way of doctors. Why? Because the outcomes might be skewed; this system doesn't work for human beings with a muscle groups that's over the average.

OK but, if we are able to't use the ones, what techniques have we left to reap our reason?

• Get out the measuring tape: right right here, you'll get your body fat percentage by way of the usage of a complicated equation concerning your weight, age, similarly to the measures from your hips, neck, waist… If you'd want to strive that approach, make it much less difficult on you and use an on-line calculator. But frankly, I'm now not a massive fan of it because of the reality, once more, the consequences is probably skewed depending for your unique morphology (huge neck, skinny waist, large hips…);

• Get yourself some calipers: need to get your numbers but don't enjoy like breaking the economic organization? For the rate of a Big Mac meal, you can purchase a couple of calipers that allows you to get the method completed. Simply comply with the suggestions which you'll locate with the tool and take measures at unique factors similar to the again, the fingers… The reliability is tremendous to 3 percentage, but that ought to give you a difficult estimate of wherein you're fame, for cheap;

• Hop on biometric scales: moreover referred to as "body fat" or "bioelectric impedance" scales, those paintings similar to your everyday scales; they are in a function to inform how an awful lot you weigh at the same time as you step on them. But, extra precious to us here, they may have a look at your body composition thru sending a contemporary thru your body to be able to deliver out the proportion of every tissue. Although a few people awesome swear through them, I'm frankly now not impressed. I discover they're too flaky in their readings because their precision can range depending at the quantity of water you're keeping, for example.

In the quit, don't move pulling your hair. Order some calipers on the Net and take a few minutes to take the measurements. It might not be the very terrific possibility however, like I said, calipers are cheap and we don't need to recognize your body fat percentage right all the way down to the very last decimal thing besides.

Now you've had been given your digits; it's time to evaluate the damage! Numbers don't lie. So, allow's man up and word wherein we're popularity.

You're over 26% body fats: sorry to break the statistics but you've been going a piece too heavy on the snacks, my friend! It's time to roll up your sleeves and get to paintings! For now, forget approximately all about getting a six-percentage… I don't want to sound like a wet blanket or lecture you however we're speakme about your health right here. Your first intention might be to go below 20% to reduce cardiovascular and one-of-a-kind related dangers.

You're among 25-18% frame fat: at this degree, you've not however lost sight of your ft however that shouldn't be prolonged in case you maintain to percent on the pounds. Your abs are although nowhere to be visible.

You're among 17-14% body fats: OK, we're slowly getting there. You don't want lots in your six-% to begin to show. This is the amount of frame fat of those who're stated to be "in form."

You're among 12-7% frame fats: brilliant, you're already pretty at the ripped aspect! Whatever it is you're doing, keep to do it because it seems to be operating. I might possibly most effective advocate you enforce the carrying sports we'll see below to in addition supply a boost to your middle. This is the variety most human beings are centered on once they're looking for to get a six-%. We'll cause for 10%, as a long way as we're concerned. You'll look extraordinary at that large variety and also you'll be capable of preserve it without too much problem.

You're beneath 6% body fats: rattling, dude! Put some clothes for your decrease lower returned; you're going to seize a chilly! This is how lean professional bodybuilders can get for a competition. It's not counseled to hold such low numbers for any term as your body desires a pleasant degree of frame fats to characteristic optimally. That's why getting so low obtained't be any of our business employer right here.

If all this speak although doesn't strike a chord and also you'd as an alternative have a visible beneficial useful resource, right right here's a chart to reveal you what each elegance looks like. As the pronouncing goes: a image is well certainly worth one thousand terms, right?

The Magic Formula

If, like we've decided an awful lot to our dismay, the usage of ourselves silly with abs carrying activities will now not be enough to pressure our abs out, we'll ought to integrate our middle education with distinctive techniques to get that body fat down.

Without going into too much element, to achieve that revel in, we'll must burn more energy than we're taking in. It's sincerely no rocket technology; it's a clean addition-subtraction operation.

Whichever street you decide to embark on, the general machine will stay same:

Abs Training + Diet + Cardio = Bell Core Fitness

Effective Workouts for Abs

Have you ever met all people who has six p.C. Abs however is pudgy everywhere else? Most probably no longer. The purpose for pointing this out is because while you do particular center strengthening physical video games, its now not without a doubt your abs that get worked on however your entire frame as well. Before shifting in the path of the exceptional exercising moves, it's far first essential to talk about the following facts: Proper Body Positioning and Developing Resistance.

Proper Body Positioning

Proper body positioning is the vital aspect to powerful core strengthening. You do not want to area vain pressure to your decrease lower again that may purpose painful injuries.

One vital right body positioning whilst you are doing floor middle strengthening sporting sports consists of well tilting your pelvis at some stage in your exercising. This is by the use of mendacity flat on the floor and then slowly arching arching your again. After that, you tilt the pinnacle part of your pelvis in advance. This positioning is known as the anterior pelvic tilt. When you waft your pelvis back off on the floor, you've got carried out the posterior pelvic tilt.

Core strengthening bodily sports in the putting feature consists of each other crucial right frame positioning. The not unusual - but incorrect - way of doing it's miles to barely arch the lower returned because the person does his placing knee or leg boom sporting activities. The higher way is to in reality spherical out the once more as you do those placing sports activities and permit the abs do all the art work.

In a nutshell, in powerful center strengthening, you have to consciously use the belly muscle mass to elevate your body at some point of these sporting sports in area of making your decrease lower returned muscle mass do it. Developing Resistance

In order to efficiently extend six percentage abs, you need to apprehend the proper amount of repetitions on the aspect of the proper type of wearing sports, otherwise you may be dropping pretty a while and electricity. The key to getting the ones abs is through manner of spending extra time on movements so as to assignment your frame even extra. A individual who does 100 crunches every day is a whole lot much less probable to expand his abs as compared to someone who does loads of big compound moves consisting of lunges, deadlifts and squats.

Core strengthening calls for approximately 10 to fifteen mins of reps 3 instances every, preferably performed after working out different muscle agencies. But in case your aim is to get abs inner 30 days, then you will need to do it 10 mins a day.

Effective Exercises for Core Strengthening

The notion of doing crunches with the useful resource of curling your top frame upwards is surely taken into consideration to be much less powerful compared to lower frame crunches. That's because of the reality the legs are heavier in comparison to your better torso. The concept is first of all lower body curl the us of americaand then upon exhaustion, you opposite to better frame curl united statessimply to finish it off.

In this section, you may be added to the top notch physical video games that you will be doing in the course of this 30-day middle strengthening software program. Work on turning into higher at them by way of way of using gradually developing the quantity and pace of the set and reps as you end up extra resistant, and shortening the rest intervals in among. And other than focusing at the belly muscles, proper middle strengthening moreover requires you to growth your decrease lower back muscle tissues and hip flexors.

But earlier than moving directly to the wearing occasions, have a examine the vain physical video games which you want to keep away from: take a seat down-u.S.With your feet being supported, device-primarily based definitely completely ab sports activities sports and twisting bodily video games, torso twists, sit down-usawith legs instantly, mendacity at once leg will increase, and striking leg will increase along side your again arched.

Moving ahead, you can now get to realise the special bodily activities that you could attention on so that you can increase your abs together with your hip flexors:

Reverse Crunches.

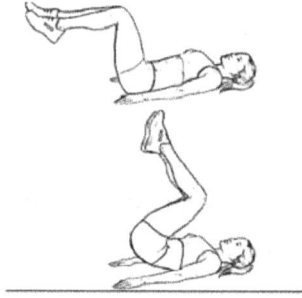

In this exercise, lie down on a mat in conjunction with your fingers going thru down on the floor next in your hips and your head and shoulders off the ground. Place your toes flat at the floor together with your knees at a 90∘ attitude. Then, slowly raise your decrease body from the floor to a crunch role the use of your ab muscle organizations and hip flexors. Avoid "swinging" or utilising momentum to do this exercise.

Ab Bicycles.

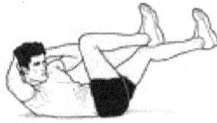

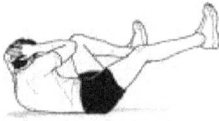

This exercising will appear like you are using a bicycle whilst in your lower lower back on the floor. First, lie down on a mat on the side of your head and shoulders slightly lifted off the floor. Bring one knee up at approximately a 90° perspective and the possibility knee barely decrease, like you're setting your ft on a motorbike's pedals. The again ought to be hunched. Your hands have to be lifted for your ears with the elbows as substantially spaced as you in all likelihood can. Begin the rep by using way of manner of "pedaling" your feet alternately, collectively together with your legs moving in a linear movement in preference to cyclical.

Ab Scissors.

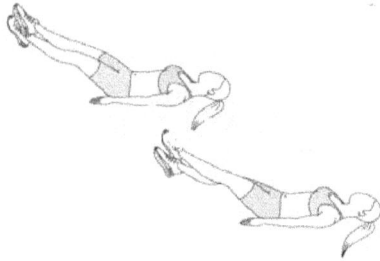

You guessed it. This exercising will flip you into a pair of human scissors, and it's going to possibly be your abs and hip flexors for you to do all of the art work. Lie in your decrease back on a mat and raise your palms instantly out over your head and your legs out, each at a 45° perspective. To carry out the pass, enhance your shoulders off whilst at the identical time bringing your legs and arms upward to barely skip each arms and legs over on top of your center.

Oblique Crunches.

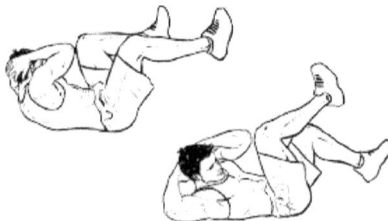

This exercise will goal your indirect muscles. Lie on the ground together collectively with your ft flat and the knees bent at approximately ninety°. Put your arms via the usage of manner of your head at the side of your elbows as extensively spaced as feasible. To perform the circulate, use your indirect muscle tissues and hip flexors to supply your right elbow to your left knee, after which repeat the alternative aspect. Make positive to carry out in a slow and stead float and to keep your crunch function for 2 counts to definitely mission the ab muscle groups.

Lying Leg Thrusts.

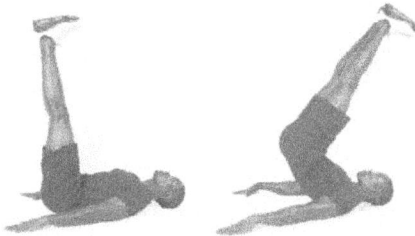

In this workout, you start by way of manner of mendacity down on a mat on the floor. The head and the shoulders have to be lifted from the ground, and your arms are faced downwards on your mat and located next on your hips. The legs want to be lifted at a 90° mindset off the ground. Then you slowly deliver your legs down but handiest half of way to the floor in region of all of the manner, at approximately a forty five° thoughts-set. Then, you bring it returned as much as the 90° attitude all yet again, and then followed through thrusting your feet upwards the usage of your ab muscle mass and hip flexors.

Decline Bench Leg Thrusts.

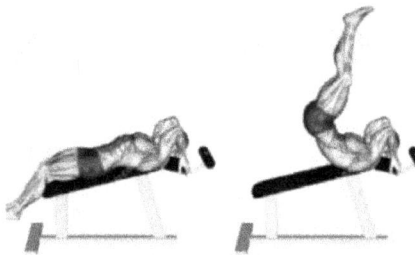

If you've got were given were given get right of get entry to to to a decline bench, then you may moreover try this exercising, it definitely is similar to the Lying Leg Thrust except its more tough. You is probably lying on the decline bench and following the identical commands from the Lying Leg Thrust except that your hands are placed, face down at the hand relaxation above your head at the decline bench.

Mountain Climber.

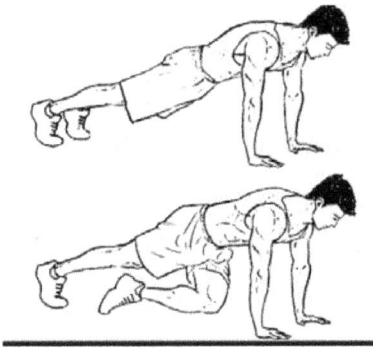

Position your arms on the ground as if you are approximately to do a push-up. Position your proper leg inward such that your knee is parallel on your chest. The left leg is stretch out inside the again of you, knee slightly bent, as in case you are approximately to move slowly. Alternate the region as speedy as you can, like you are hiking a mountain. Make positive to have interaction the abs in the route of this workout.

Mountain Jumper.

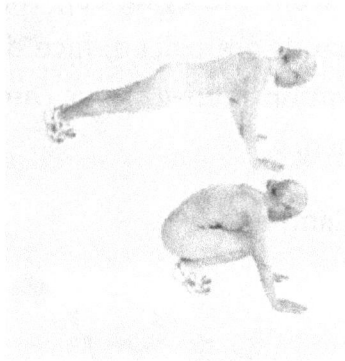

This is a extra intense exchange of mountain climber wherein you will start with each legs stretched out within the back of you as if you are going to do a push-up, and then "jumping" to a characteristic with the knees brought near your elbows. Don't forget about to engage your ab muscle corporations as properly.

Hanging Leg Raises (with rounded lower lower back and shoulders). Grip a pull-up bar collectively with your hands parallel in conjunction with your shoulders. The knees should be immediately or barely bent. With your abs and hip flexors, pull your legs as a great deal as the pull-up bar or as a long way as you may circulate. Ensure which you do the ones bodily games with a rounded lower back and shoulders in choice to arching your again. Beginners or humans with shoulder problems can use elbow straps with this exercising.

Hanging Knee Raises (with rounded once more and shoulders). This exercising is much like the Hanging Leg Raises however this time your knees are completely bent. With your abs and hip flexors, enhance your knees up to your chest. The purpose why this change got here to be is as it minimizes the load which you are lifting.

You can pick out out out any time of the day that is maximum reachable on the way to do your workout. Just ensure to do it frequently. Some humans like to do it early within the morning, even as others do it within the overdue afternoon. Don't neglect to have your pre-exercise and post-exercise food so you obtained't come to be binge ingesting at the stop of your education. Your pre-exercising snacks want to be crafted from protein-packed whole foods inclusive of nuts, seeds and a hardboiled egg. Your pre-exercise snacks should be low in fats and excessive in nutrients and minerals which encompass a banana or an apple.

Chapter 4: WAYS TO LOSE BELLY FAT

If you commit each day to normal exercising and right vitamins, you may in no way want to stand in the the front of the reflect and ask yourself, "Do I need to take off a few weight?" Once we come to this hassle, it is late and the answer is pretty clean. We live in an age wherein it isn't always sufficient to be in proper shape, we want to be in great form!

Of direction, this is not so smooth to gain - at least no longer all of the time. However, summer season is generally "throughout the nook" and anyone want to get into shape for summer season. There isn't any time-venerated answer for putting off fats from the stomach. There are masses of solutions to this hassle, however normally if you examine the ones 10 guidelines, you'll do well.

1.Eat greater protein.

If you idea that this does not ought to be mentioned, you're wrong − it's pretty the opportunity. In addition to being very healthy to your frame, proteins preserve muscular tissues, at the identical time as diet and make sure which you burn no longer some thing but undesirable fat.

2.Compete

You won't ought to go out on degree in Speedo trunks and pose inside the the front of 800 humans, but you want to make demanding situations for yourself each time you enter the fitness center. Last time you have got been doing squats 4 series, now you have got have been given finished 5 series. You labored rapid on foot at an mind-set of 8 stages, nowadays growth the angle to ten stages and walk for 10 mins longer.

three.Throw Away Carbs

The high-quality tactic is to put off all resources of digestible carbohydrates inside the complete weeks at the start of the healthy dietweight-reduction plan. This device is so clean, and so it really works nicely whilst implemented, nearly, tremendous. Just take into account your green greens - broccoli and lettuce are your remarkable friends.

4.Don't skip food.

It's splendid how many human beings nowadays pass meals, all hoping to burn fat quicker. This will not most effective sluggish down the approach of burning fat, but will probable accelerate the approach of burning your muscle groups. This is the instant at the same time as operating out starts offevolved to feel especially tough.

five.Drink extra water.

Drink one glass of water before the meal and one glass 1/2 of an hour after the meal. The glass earlier than meals will lessen your urge for meals, and the handiest after will keep you hydrated at some level in the day.

6.Avoid snacks

That seductive lady voice on TV searching out to persuade you that their snacks are tasty, and that you could advantage the right form without dieting, is telling lies! It's higher to eat a cardboard field in which the snacks are packaged – it has more treasured nutrients than those snacks. Stick to natural meals you in my view make.

7.Do Interval Training

There are masses of studies that show that interval schooling is better to put off fats than the traditional aerobic schooling.

eight.Go thru foot.

Whenever you have got were given the possibility to transport far taking walks use it! In this manner, you'll growth the overall type of energy you spend at some stage within the day, and I am fine that you will encounter some vintage buddies who you haven't visible in some time at the same time as on foot to locations.

9.Chew slower.

People in recent times stay faster and consequently eat faster. But that does not propose that meals is digested quicker. Half-digested meals is in the belly, then gets within the intestines and in the end it in fact gets thrown away. So, we've were given a great deal less food inside the body, the lots lots less power inside the machine and lots less protein within the muscle tissues. Just terrific situations for slowing metabolism and developing fatter.

10. Use a scale in preference to the reflect.

Keep the dimensions inside the the front of the reflect. So each time you step on the size and be conscious that the pointer is not moved you appearance inside the replicate and take a look at your self to look if your stomach is asking thinner.

Even if you exercise loads the difficulty above the waist remains not what you want. What drives you crazy the most is when the stomach fat receives poured over slowly on the equal time as you take a seat down. All you need is a extremely good flat stomach on the seaside. Well, then have a observe those recommendations and attempt to exercising them as soon as possible.

You need to keep in mind biking and exclusive aerobic activities. Cycling is one of the first-rate strategies to put off the fat pads throughout the waist.

Simply on foot or the usage of the motorbike will now not show actual brief results, it's far higher to run at durations. This schooling will assist in eliminating fats across the belly (examined). You specify periods and pace, but be cautious no longer to spare yourself too much from running out difficult.

Exercises for More Visible Muscle Tone

In addition to strolling and cycling, the first-class recommendation is that you workout your abs, however additionally do carrying sports activities for the back of the body (the decrease decrease lower back and buttocks). By education these physical sports activities, you can get leaner and get tighter frame shape. Do now not pass the exercising for the once more of your frame whilst you do the abs carrying sports.

Also, don't avoid going to fitness center. Push extra hard and hit massive weights. The extra you lift, the extra muscle you may assemble. The more muscle agencies you've got the quicker your metabolism can be. Remember muscle tissue burns more calories period, whether or not at rest or doing an hobby.

Remember that neither hard cardio nor spending hours in fitness center will help you lose belly fat if you don't accurate your weight-reduction plan. Diet is the most important issue for weight reduction and getting 6 % abs! Start making adjustments on your healthy eating plan.

Common Myths Associated with Abs

There is too much incorrect information approximately burning fat and building muscle. While there's no right or wrong manner to get a ripped body, some strategies are extra effective than others. So being aware of them will certainly assist satisfy your choice to get a washboard belly.

1.Some guys are born with six percentage abs

Busted: Some men have a better metabolism in assessment to others, which guarantees that they do no longer need to paintings as tough as others to get a ripped body. Lowering your stomach fat thru a healthful dietary and exercising recurring will assist you get the favored frame.

Chapter 5: Squat Basics

Our first trouble in 'Routine List' may be the 'Squat'. Unlike many humans assume, this time period is not concerning this regarded expertise of the clinching down movement sample and getting lower lower back up without or with weight, regularly seen. In this case, I talk over with this frequently known as 'Asian squat' or 'Deep Squat'. This one is a complete clinched, low gait and knees honestly bent, resting squat role.

In many Asian international locations like Thailand, China, Indonesia and Malaysia to call a few, the 'squat' continues to be a function very frequently used to rest, take a look at, do laundry or even wait, rather than fame. Many public lavatories have pans which makes it obligatory for human beings to have the potential to relaxation in this characteristic. The motive for it moreover stands for hygienic and sanitary capabilities. How special is it from the western worldwide, proper? Well, wager what? People in the Eastern worldwide are one step ahead with this one. But now not all is out of region, for the reason that masses people have been able to examine, watch or possibly travel to Eastern nations and undertake practices to rehabilitate our our our bodies in the direction of this critical position.

As youngsters, low gait positions together with the 'squat' are available and accessible without even thinking about it. I guess next time you'll be at a park or truely at home looking your youngsters flow and locomote at the ground, you'll be aware about their potential on getting into and coming out of these positions. They don't even think about it as a completely unique device or stressful sample, because of the reality it's far 2nd nature to them. The mistake is that after developing up, we lose it due to the fact we are knowledgeable that 'normal relaxation feature' is thru sitting on a chair.

The unfortunate reality is that our frame has a 'use it or lose it' form of technique. Which manner that for the purpose that we don't employ this feature, our joints, decrease body mobility and joint capability to build up the place is out of place, by the point we end up adults. With that come digestive issues, lower decrease once more pain and greater illnesses. Speaking of digestion, many western groups that realise the blessings of this role have started out out out selling and selling benches or 'steps' which is probably to be positioned beneath your feet as a way to emulate the 'squat' position while sitting on a rest room. This allows bowel actions, reduces constipation, alleviates digestive tract issues & aligns your colon. On the alternative hand, talking of the manner important it's far to domesticate & maintain our verbal exchange with the ground, a Brazilian health practitioner even created a take a look at this is composed in getting down and coming decrease lower back up, with little to no assist so that it will diploma your health and sturdiness. These smooth however inexperienced actions are via the usage of way of a ways one of the most underrated abilties.

OK! I firmly be given as true with we've got understood what the issues are and the damage it has prompted to so plenty folks, however sufficient is enough. Now that we've lengthy long beyond through the horrible statistics, permit's leap into the great things! The maximum fine part of this is that EVERYONE is capable of restoration this problem with the aid of rehabilitating their our our bodies to the 'Squat' position. With dedication, achievement is form of a hundred% guaranteed and you will then be rewarded with a present day, resilient and capable body.

Here are a few tips that you could observe to take manage of your fitness and get again at the proper direction. For first timers, I might also advocate you've got got somewhere to maintain onto earlier than obtaining the location, due to the fact you would possibly fall once more due to loss of mobility. This can be a bar, a put up or some thing that you could rely upon and will useful aid your body weight. Stand shoulder width aside, your feet ought to barely be pointing outwards, in a forty five diploma mind-set. We want on the manner to get down into an 'ass to grass' deep squat, flat footed as lots as feasible. In order to carry out it efficaciously, it'll require ankle and hip mobility.

If you are beginning with this, I ought to especially propose having a higher platform which incorporates a e-book, small dumbbells or any item positioned underneath your heels to elevate them. It alleviates the pressure at the ankles and optimizes higher consequences, at the same time as starting off. Also, the magic trick to achieve success is to divide it sluggish inside the squat in small sections, within the route of the day. I may recommend starting up with 10-15 mins every day, divided in small quantities of 10,20 or 30 seconds till you whole the time encouraged. It is normal to feel a bit dizzy at times while getting back up. The purpose being that our body is honestly compressed even as in the characteristic, which prevents the blood from flowing well, on the equal time as not accustomed. Consistency and exercising will necessarily get you rid of those discomforts. After ONLY 30 consecutive days, your frame could have transformed and tailored! Afterwards, the time needed to maintain this mobility is nearly shortened to 1/2 of of of it.

Recap :

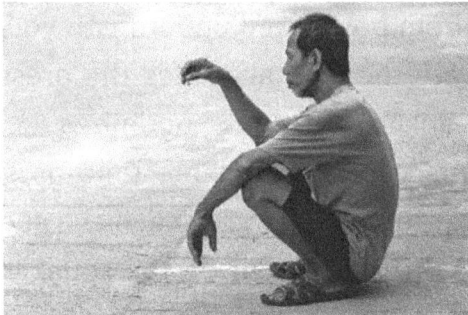

Stand shoulder width aside

•Point toes outwards, in a 45 degree angle

•Fold down right into a flat footed 'ass to grass' deep squat position

•If vital, area item underneath heels for ankles comfort

•Divide some time in small portions of 10,20 or 30 seconds till accomplishing 10-15 mins every day, fashionable time.

•Commit for 30 consecutive days and REAP THE REWARDS!

Chapter 6: Passive Hang

Next off, I would like to introduce you to the 'passive dangle'. It is regularly known as the 'lifeless hold'. Just like primates, we as human beings have the utter necessity to 'maintain'. Unlike monkeys, there not is the need to climb a tree to pick out up a fruit or brachiate and swing to move round in place. Since our hands, shoulders and scapulas had been designed to accomplish that, setting is like our 'cat stretch' , the way we growth the body completely and generate this opposite effect of compression on the frame. In fact, it is able to additionally be perceived as self-chiropractor because it lets in you to regain shoulder mobility, brushes off neck pain, creates place in amongst vertebrae or even relieves your lower lower returned.

Our our bodies are suffering from gravity, static positions and consequently backbone constriction. The lack of time spent 'striking' generates pain, calcification and absence of overhead palms mobility. Studies have confirmed that eighty% of Americans can be by means of decrease back ache at least as soon as in their whole existence. In 2017, a have a have a look at confirmed that decrease back pain modified into indexed due to the fact the LEADER in cause of incapacity in the WORLD. These numbers are horrifying, aren't they? Just just like the squat, passive setting doesn't get referred to enough almost about well being, ache unfastened frame workout or without a doubt every day conduct. But fortuitously for you, after having this statistics to your toolbox, you'll be a part of the small percent of people who no longer be afflicted by way of once more ache. I'm absolutely happy to be sharing this, due to the truth I understand for sure that it's miles a activity changer. When addressed and practiced properly, the advantages are lifestyles converting!

Here's how you could get it going with this 'hack'. First, it is recommended to have a pull up bar hooked up to your door frame or everywhere in your private home. Such matters will sell greater time setting and help you version. When it involves the act of setting, we need to have a business enterprise maintain near via putting the palm of our hand on the bar and wrapping our hands spherical it. At the pinnacle of the bar, we are capable of have our arms from pinky to index wrapped round it, and our thumb will pass below the bar and meet on the opportunity element with the 4 palms, as if you have been grabbing a stick, firmly.

After that, we are able to slowly release tension until we obtain maximum body extension, by means of manner of manner of getting our fingers directly, allowing our ribcage to launch. Shoulders need to be touching our ears, or at least very close to them. Sense your top frame and launch scapula, again, ribs and abs anxiety to optimize the drill. If you are a amateur, I might also advocate having 1 or 2 feet at the floor, that way you can step by step dose the frame weight for your forearms and palms. The aim being to attain entire frame release, in the end. Similar to the squat, we want to divide our putting in small 10, 20 or 30 2nd components and growth to 5 mins every day. Incorporate it for 30 consecutive days. I can not endorse this one enough! Trust the method and it's going to trade your existence!

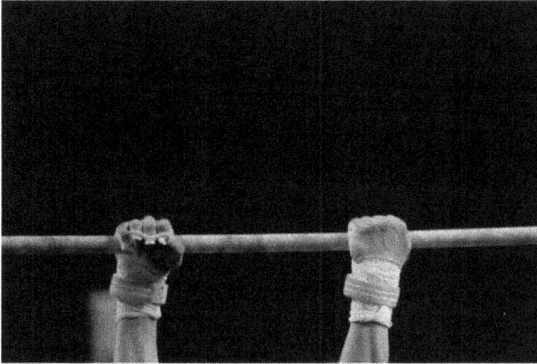

Recap :

•Install a pull up bar

•Place palm of hand on bar shoulder width apart and wrap hands spherical firmly

•Release entire upper frame anxiety till shoulders contact ears

•If a novice, contact the ground with toes which will often release body weight

•Divide it gradual in small portions of 10,20 or 30 seconds till carrying out 5 minutes every day, regular time.

•Commit for 30 consecutive days and LIVE FREE OF BACK PAIN!

Chapter 7: Shake it Off!

Up subsequent in line, I'd need to introduce you to the 'shaking'. When we pay attention this word, we will be predisposed to consider vibrating, agitating and jiggling. As said inside the subtitle, I will percentage the importance of 'Shaking it off', why animals shake and the way it's far beneficial for us human beings.

As modern human beings, the act of shaking off isn't very not unusual to us and can also be visible as 'uncommon' to appearance someone shaking. But, the question proper right here is, why do animals shake? I'd like for us to take a fellow species, very near us and international broadly recognized with the useful resource of Mr. King Frederick of Prussia as : A Man's Best Friend. As you guessed, we're talking approximately DOGS. I anticipate you robotically make the correlation of a dog shaking off from head to toe, proper? As we may also moreover recognize, puppies often shake while finishing their swim, after waking up or finishing their grooming.

But, if we take a better look, similarly they do at one-of-a-type times of the day. The purpose within the lower back of this instinctive 'shaking' is as it eliminates trauma, helps them launch tension or even receives rid of pressure. Dogs perform it right after a hug, a cuddle or a caress. Many additionally carry out it after coming down from the veterinarian's table, as though they had been casting off the stressful and unpleasant 2d they were encountering at that particular moment. Whether we recognize it or not, shaking has been, is and could all the time be an instinctive 'pattern' that animals use in the equal fashion that puppies do. Although it has in no way been validated to them with the useful useful resource of any manner, shape or form, they employ this notable device intuitively, every time they experience the want for it.

That being understood, we apprehend that 'shaking' is a effective, beneficial and key practice that is frequently now not sorted or overseen through the usage of us human beings. Although we do no longer perform as '2d nature' like animals, we from time to time do while we experience it's cold or at the same time as we taste something that is very bitter. I can nearly assure you can relate to the type of moments on the same time as you placed yourself shaking for a brief 2d. If we dig a chunk deeper, we can understand that when this shaking, our frame releases pressure and tension from the incident encountered, proper? That evaluation necessarily tells us a few difficulty : Our device is aware of about it and it is however alive somewhere indoors parents! Isn't that correct facts? The conflict isn't out of place and we aren't too far from getting decrease lower back at the proper music. This is a fantastic and effective 'hack' that may best do right for us current-day humans, residing in a stressful society. The advantages of shaking may be with pain consolation, harm prevention and blood go with the go with the flow optimization, to call some. This method of exercising has been seen in order fields which includes yoga, for instance. It is also used for the reason of loosening up, relieving pressure and waking up the frame.

Here is a fixed of steerage to be able to begin your adventure inside the path of 'shaking it off'!. First, you may stand stall and immediately, barefoot, shoulder width aside and looking within the path of the the the front or together with your eyes closed. Have a comfortable jaw, allow the mouth to softly open if desired and make sure not to preserve the breathing. Arms down, fun your bum and your belly, grounded flat footed and really tiny moderate knee bent. The motive within the back of it's far to launch rigidity, loosen up the pelvic ground and hips in order for the electricity to skip thru the body. You need to not straighten, nor bend the knees to sense anxiety on the legs. As tons as we want to enjoy grounded, there desires to be an hobby closer to not compressing too much the higher body. To prevent it from going on, we're able to remember that we've 2 palms slightly pulling our head up within the direction of the sky, stretching our neck and straightening our again. REMEMBER, the posture ought to be of little to no tension the least bit.

Once that is addressed, we are able to very barely bend our knees and straighten them, repetitively to initiate the movement. At the equal time, we are capable of bring our heels and drop them backtrack intently, to generate vibration with the impact. It is crucial to drop down as prescribed for the frame to feel the vibration that starts offevolved offevolved offevolved from the feet and goes all of the way to the pinnacle. Understanding that, we are capable of gently repeat the exercise and find rhythm to supply a slight and non-stop 'rebound' impact in among the start and the forestall factor. You must sense the complete body vibrating from the indoors (torso) towards the out of doors (limbs). The magic takes place even as we input in the 'shaking america', no longer permitting the frame to stay static, then slowly check our frame and launch anxiety within the shoulders, elbows, wrists, abs, glutes, and even the face, on the same time as in the nation.

My advice is to have a three-five minute shake, each day. Once the concept of freeing anxiety and shaking is owned, it is transferable to different additives of the body. For instance, allow's have a look at it for the wrist. First, we are able to have our arm clearly 'useless', no tension via way of any way. We will rotate our wrist as despite the fact that we had been turning a door knob, then gently discover rhythm and have a examine the bouncing sensation. Once the sample is determined, we test our whole arm and release our palms, wrist, forearm, bicep, tricep, shoulder and VOILA! Another detail to take into account is that the ones 'rebounding' factors have to no longer be too a ways from every exclusive nor the sample too lengthy, due to the truth we need to control and traumatic the body as low as feasible and 'jiggle' our our our bodies with little to no tension the least bit. The same technique is applicable for anywhere else on the frame. Since I want to help my fellow readers to manual themselves a hint bit, I will help you with a list of body components that you may strive your 'shaking' method with :

•Head (up and down vertically or side to aspect, horizontal sample)

•knees (mild up and down rebounds or aspect to side sample)

•elbows (up and down or the the the front to again pattern)

•Wrists (up and down or rotating as defined previously)

Like many things, the fundamentals want to be truely understood and done effectively so you can shift within the direction of extra complicated degrees. There are NO RULES aside from that, due to this that that as soon as we discover a 'shakeable' sample, WE REAP OUT THE BENEFITS! It's as clean as it receives. Now, some different layer I have to issue out and deal with is the way to get out of the so-known as 'shaking nation'. I trust this element to be as crucial and useful as a few other thing of the routine, given that it is while we enjoy and acquire the well-deserved endorphins.

How to get again to motionlessness is as easy as very slowly reducing speed and shortening the length of the sample we're acting until we achieve complete stillness. This approach must take you about 10 seconds, type of. When getting there, we must continue to be although for at least a minute and SENSE the vibrations, revel in the blood flowing and the softness that it produces. Shaking is so powerful and regenerative that I especially suggest you contain it into your day by day normal. Like all matters, workout and consistency will simplest propel you inside the route of a higher know-how and nicely finished practice. Like all preceding 'hacks', I'd quite advise you commit for at the least 1 month, as a way to enjoy, experience and revel in the advantages that it offers.

Recap :

• Choose a body detail

• Identify the sample's begin and quit problem

• Generate the 'rebound sensation' in amongst factors

• Scan your frame and launch all strain,

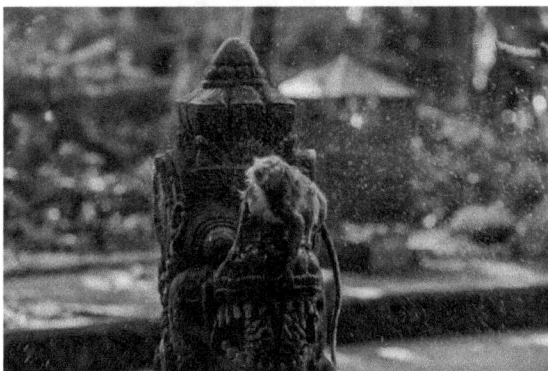

anxiety or useless strain

• Enter into the shaking kingdom for 3-five mins

• Reduce velocity step by step till attaining whole stillness

• Remain immobile and experience the internal 'vibrations' for at least 1 minute

•Commit for 30 consecutive days and LIVE A STRESS FREE LIFE!

Chapter 8: Spinal Waves

This one is certainly one of my favorites and that is why I saved it for the remaining. One of the maximum powerful workouts you may put into effect into your each day life is the 'Spinal Wave'. Many practices and teachers have placed this effective device and it has advanced the lives of all of us embracing it and integrating it into their every day to-do-listing.

Our spine consists of 24 vertebrae, stacked on pinnacle of every extraordinary. It is the center of our complete body and it's far what permits us to transport. Almost every part of the frame may be taken off, but so long as we have were given the spine, we will always have the capability to be in movement. All moves originate from the spine, while you consider that it's far our middle. No frame detail may be moved without the spine to be affected. It can be perceived because the 'for each motion there may be a response' analogy. If you circulate your huge toe, it robotically affects the foot, which translates into the leg, that is related to the glute and it is glued to the decrease part of the spine. Same detail is going for the arm, if a finger is moved, it is translated into the forearm which then influences the elbow and the scapula, that is related to the higher backbone. Within the human frame, there may be no such factor because of the reality the isolation of a movement. Every component is tied up and correlated all together. Extremities (limbs) are interlaced with middle (backbone). It is important for us to understand those factors earlier than diving deeper into the problem count number. Why? Because while we apprehend the bigger photo and complexity of the problem, we will deal with the fundamentals, the chore and the muse of it, which in the end fixes the entire engine.

That being stated, allow's jump into extra realistic statistics. Our backbone have become designed to transport in plenty of severa components collectively with : compressing, extending, twisting and bending, to call some. The extra we cultivate them, the greater resilient, tailored and supple the spine can be. The motive within the lower back of many all over again hassle troubles is the lack of complexity into the spine. Our cutting-edge-day manner of existence does now not provide us with any tool nor indicates any first rate habits to prevent the ones issues. Like we said earlier, a massive percentage of the human populace suffers from again ache, but unfortunately we most effective pay attention about magic tablets or static postures to evolve to as a manner to restore the problem, which in the end most effective is a short time period repair. As anybody recognize, if we're to do some thing, we should do it properly.

For example, allow's take one of the topics that are not honestly addressed and misunderstood in my opinion. That is the POSTURE. Like we can also apprehend, present day-day global human beings spend quite some time working at a table, within the the front of a laptop. That entails a static posture which may be complex, however allow's no longer lose our focus at the priority here. The truth of having to work at a desk 'well' implies a positive 'proper posture'. Well, I am right here to inform you that there may be no such issue as a proper posture. Based on the truth that our spine changed into designed to move in complex strategies, we want to rehabilitate our spine stressors and therefore make it greater resilient to as many 'postures' as feasible. Now, permit's be honest, sitting at once at the identical time as jogging on a desk can actually be higher than going for walks with a hunched once more.

One of the primary topics to address is : Resiliency. At a completely younger age, much like many joints, our spine has the capability to transport in masses of methods. The elasticity of the kid's spine is impressive. The cause being that they haven't but accompanied a each day habitual that doesn't contain 'transferring'. Of direction, children do it in an subconscious manner in view that they will be in the direction of the instinctive supply of humanity. Their actions and strategies of shifting are only driven via their instinct, it really is notable. Although us adults do now not have this instinct mounted in that regard, we are able to in truth declare our backbone vocabulary returned and attach our problems. The more vocabulary there can be, the greater movement interest you will get to experience. And this is at the same time as we dive into the actual art work. Because there may be no factor of getting a senseless workout, without feeling, information and sensing what is going on interior of you. We regularly pay attention human beings announcing : "Listen in your frame". The actual query is : "Do you have were given sufficient vocabulary to pay attention, recognize and cope with what your body is telling you?". That is what I am eager to provide to you.

Here is how you can begin building a vocabulary inside the route of a painless body, thru 'spinal waves'. First, we are able to stand tall half of of a foot duration within the front of a wall. This wall goes to be used as a reference thing to 'articulating' our spine nicely. Then, we are able to list all elements of the frame which may be to be used to generate the 'wave'. These are : the nostril, chin, chest, ribs, belly and pelvis. We have to make sure to simplest touch the wall with one part of the frame, then update it with the following one in line. Once you've reached the very last aspect being the pelvis, you come to the first issue being the nostril. Make positive to genuinely contact the wall with all people factor and take a one-2d pause on each phase. It is obligatory to memorize this collection for max notable outcomes. One aspect that may be executed is to mention it on your head, while going via every and every aspect. Practice more than one times an afternoon for at least 3-five minutes, with the intention to accumulate a fluid pattern. With time, you'll be capable of back down of the wall and carry out it fluidly, with out pausing in every segment. This on my own will disregard stagnation, pains, discomforts and rubdown or awaken factors of your body that had been snoozing and forgotten for years.

By unlocking those moves and regaining backbone mobility, you will then be able to find out, bypass and interpret new movement styles that possibly weren't available within the past. That is while we begin developing this 'vocabulary' this is extraordinarily beneficial to 'body map' and cope with the aches felt on your torso and higher body. Making it a ordinary will facilitate all backbone moves, on the way to then translate into the rest of the body. As we stated, the backbone impacts each part of the body, and vice versa. The advantages of releasing our backbone actions is that it will beautify the potential to throw, dance, stability, locomote, LIVE! As the call of the e-book says, those noticeably outstanding physical activities 'hacks' are suitable for beginners. But, allow's no longer overlook about them for one 2d. All of those equipment also can increase our overall performance in special specific or extra specialized fields, whilst you endure in mind that those home device cope with the human, which stands in advance than a few trouble.

In one-of-a-kind phrases, first there can be the human, most effective then can we emerge as a expert.

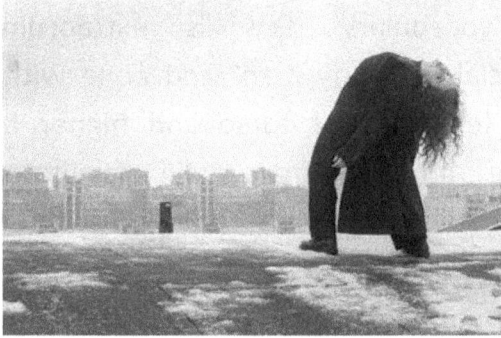

Recap :

•Stand stall, 1/2 foot length inside the the front of the wall

•Perform nostril to pelvis collection inside the maximum articulated manner possible

•Say the series to your head to facilitate memorizing the pattern

•Repeat the gathering continuously until engaging in fluidity

•Perform for 3-five minutes, a couple of instances every day

•Commit for 30 consecutive days and REJUVENATE YOUR SPINE!

Information is essential, which I apprehend for a fact that you apprehend this. If no longer, you wouldn't have purchased this e-book. I am so satisfied you got to this point of the e-book, due to the fact the ones existence changing gadget will all the time be stored in you and you are on the verge of becoming a one in all a kind person!

Chapter 9: Environmental Adaptations & Behaviors

Lastly, I would like that will help you shift your interest to brilliant factors, to facilitate the incorporation of these behavior, exercises and 'hacks' into your every day lifestyles. My first idea is probably to install a pull up bar in a door frame which you pass through very often, at domestic. The motive being that it'll incentivize you to comprehend often without even questioning an excessive amount of of putting a time for exercise inside the route of the day, but as an alternative, make it a each day 2d nature obligation like brushing your enamel, consuming espresso or every other each day dependancy. If you take location to make money working from home or simply throughout regular time, take 'putting breaks'! Those little each day conduct can alternate your complete frame exponentially, if done every day. That's a 'HACK' right there.

Secondly, in phrases of the squat function I ought to recommend you to be the 'bizarre' character. Yes, as you honestly examine.

Whenever you have got spare time, acquire the position! When eating espresso, reading, waiting for the bus, or deciding on up items from the floor. This will make it extra interesting and make it experience an lousy lot a good deal less as a duty, however extra every exceptional static function, it is the case, in the end.

Thirdly, start growing this frame attention and spotting whilst the frame is longing for oscillating the spine with a few waves, or some 'putting'. Being capable of come to be aware of and take note of the body is with the aid of an extended manner a bargain more powerful than a few thing else, due to the reality after rehabilitating your frame the first rate way a good way to hold it supple, oily and mobile is with the useful resource of recognizing the signs and symptoms and signs and symptoms that it gives to you. The satisfactory way to transport approximately that is to create what I like to name a 'Life Practice'. This way which you are diligent and aware of the art work that needs to be finished but the ones behavior and sporting sports end up part of your regular everyday existence. That manner you do no longer constantly experience the need to set time apart or go to the health club (in case you're now not used to). Since you presently have those equipment, you'll almost in no manner be in need of some thing or anybody else to push aside your aches and discomforts.

Chapter 10: Introduction to Fitness

Thank you for buying this ebook! By looking for this ebook, you have got confirmed hobby in turn ing into a higher, more healthy version of your self. Millions of humans start a ultra-modern-day in shape journey each and every three hundred and sixty 5 days, and you can be certainly one in every of them in no time.

Over the very last decade, fitness has come to be a real worldwide phenomenon. Every 12 months human beings enthusiastically start hitting the health club, taking walks or ingesting healthful. When humans consider health, they usually recollect hundred+ pounds men lifting heavy weights and being mean to the modern-day day weaker guys inside the health club, but that's far from the reality. Fitness shouldn't be about the fact that you're capable of deadlift over four hundred lbs or being capable of do 50 pullups.

A lot of people don't go to the gym due to the reality they fear they will no longer be widespread for what how they look. Just consider that each single one of the humans inside the gym commenced off just like you, everyone commenced off lifting the slight weights with a crappy form and in the occasion that they've been capable of turn out to be what they will be in recent times, you could do it as properly.

In this e-book, you will be guided via the fundamentals of health little by little. These fundaments can be carried out whether you're a newbie, an intermediate or a complex lifter. You can be added to all of the essential subjects inside the fitness corporation, from running out to vitamins, to the issues people normally normally have a tendency to miss which embody electricity of will and what to do out of doors of the health club.

Chapter 11: Exercise

One of the crucial detail elements of health is exercise. Exercising is to be had in lots of bureaucracy and brands. Whether you want to run, swim, cycle or go with the flow the fitness center, exercise is the foundation of creating a extra healthy manner of existence and begin your health journey. Even despite the fact that this ebook is based spherical health and taking walks out inside the fitness center, you may but observe all of the cited tips and pointers to some different shape of workout.

There are methods to exercise at a everyday health club. You can do a ordinary workout, powerlifting, CrossFit, High-Intensity Interval Training or many one in every of a kind sorts of exercising. Even despite the fact that there are many techniques to workout they all begin with the equal principle, start off slowly. Every fitness teach will teach you the equal precept, form before weights. Often novices, or perhaps advanced lifters, visit the gym and begin 'ego lifting' which means that

that human beings will use heavier weights to look robust, however their form will undergo. Not high-quality does this save you you from gaining strength, but you can additionally even get severely injured if you do not use proper techniques.

When you start operating out at a gymnasium, it's far critical to start off with studying the proper techniques. It is commonly encouraged that you ask a more expert buddy or a gym worker to help you out and teach you a manner to do every exercise. You can start out via using doing loose weight or device physical sports. Both loose weight and machine exercise have benefits and drawbacks. Free weight physical games are greater tough to perform nicely, especially on the same time as you are a newbie, however they'll growth your profits. Machine wearing occasions are an amazing manner to learn how to use proper techniques in advance than you skip right away to free weight exercising no matter the reality that they will restriction your benefit within the beginning.

When you are a amateur on the health club, it's far vital to begin with lighter weights. Your muscle will have to get used to weight education, and it is less complicated to have a look at right form while you are using lighter weights. When you are able to perform every exercising properly, you could begin growing the weights little by little.

Each exercising is composed out of a positive quantity of units and repetitions, additionally called reps. Sets are the sort of times you do every workout; repetitions are the form of instances you repeat the movement. The form of reps may be broken down into three sections. The first section is among 1 and six reps, on every occasion you train 1-6 reps you're using maximal attempt, the 1-6 rep range is often used by powerlifters and people trying to interrupt their personal information. The second segment is amongst 6 and 12 reps. Training amongst 6 and 12 reps is most often related to building muscle. The final rep phase is 12 reps and above. The 12+ rep variety is idea for muscle staying electricity, however it although builds muscle. Beginners regularly start off with 15 reps constant with devices, three sets every exercising. When time progresses human beings seeking to assemble muscle must pass for six to 12 reps, while humans in search of to lose fat want to stay within the 12+ rep range. Of route, each rep variety can be used for distinctive functions. Some of the super bodybuilders of all time used a higher rep variety to collect muscle, and some people out of place an entire lot of fats with the aid of using using decrease rep tiers. It's recommended to discern out what suits your body the extremely good.

Of direction, lifting is not the exceptional way you could workout in a fitness center. Whenever you enter a gymnasium, you can see more than one cardiovascular machines. A lot of people use aerobic as a warm up, or as a cooldown on the result in their workout. Even despite the reality that aerobic is an wonderful way to construct your condition, it's also a generally used approach to lose fats. For people attempting to find to lose fat, ordinary cardio appears to be the higher choice. People that are looking for to gather muscle at the identical time as losing fat frequently use HIIT, High-Intensity Interval Training. As the call shows, HIIT education approach doing brief intervals of maximal attempt cardio located by way of long rest durations. For example, you do 15 to 30 seconds of maximal effort taking walks on the treadmill located with the useful resource of the use of 1 to 2 minutes recovery repeating the same cycle more than one times.

When you start training, you have to workout approximately 2 or three times each week. You must have as a minimum 48 hours amongst every whole body exercise, so your body has time to get better. Beginners need to start off with a complete-body ordinary so their body can get used to training. Depending on how a good deal time you have got were given, it's endorsed to do one exercise for all people part, if you don't have the time to do one exercise for each frame element you ought to use compound sports. Compound sports activities sports are physical activities that hit multiple muscle companies immediately. The maximum not unusual compound sporting sports are the bench press, which hits the chest, shoulders, and triceps, the seated row, which hits your lower lower back, biceps, and the lowest of your shoulders and traps, and in the long run the squat, which hits your entire legs and your middle. For demonstration functions, two entire-frame carrying activities can be listed beneath.

Full-frame workout 1: Warm up five-10 minutes of biking, (device) bench press three units of 15 reps, seated decrease again row 3 gadgets of 15 reps, leg press or (tool squat) 3 devices of 15 reps, crunches three units of 15 reps, optionally to be had five-10 mins treadmill.

Chapter 12: Nutrition

Nutrition is in reality as, if not more important than exercising. Nutrition is your frame's gasoline, and it's miles important to understand the manner to well get your nutrients in case you need to transform your body.

A lot of human beings partner nutrients with strength, and regardless of the fact that counting power is a wonderful indicator of tracking your vitamins, it's far handiest scratching the floor. Eating 200 electricity nicely virtually worth of bird breast is healthier than ingesting hundred power well properly well worth of fries, despite the reality which you devour the same amount of strength the impact it has on your body is way distinct. That's why a number of athletes don't actually tune their strength, but also their macronutrients.

The three macronutrients, also called macros, are carbohydrates, protein, and fats. Whenever you take a look at the nutrients records on a product, you may find out all the resources as cited above and further. Each this sort of three macronutrients has their advantages and also you need to take word of all of them in case you need to transform your body well.

Carbohydrates are the 'gasoline' of your body. They offer you with the electricity to feature on a each day basis. Without the proper amounts of carbohydrates, your frame may have to begin the use of fat and protein as electricity resources. As an instance, some carbohydrate assets may be listed under.

•Bananas

•Oats

•(Sweet) potatoes

•(Brown) rice

The subsequent macronutrient is protein. Protein is the macronutrient that grows your muscles. Protein includes amino acids; there are 22 amino acids, 8 of which can be referred to as 'critical amino acids' due to this you have to eat those amino acids when you recollect that your frame can't produce them on its very own. It's important to consume more than one resources of protein to ensure you're consuming all the critical amino acids. How an awful lot protein you need to eat is predicated upon in your dreams and your body weight. The commonplace guy have to consume around fifty six grams of protein an afternoon, on the same time as the common woman have to consume 46 grams of protein a day. However, in case your purpose is to assemble muscle, it's miles recommended to consume 1 gram of protein in keeping with pound of bodyweight/2.2 grams of protein regular with kg of body weight. If you're seeking to gather muscle, you need to consume 20 to twenty-5 grams of protein each 3 hours. The most not unusual manner of consuming protein is animal protein, which moreover gives the body with all the vital amino acids. However, it's though possible to devour sufficient protein in case you're a vegetarian or vegan. Of path, you may also consume protein through protein powders and extraordinary dietary supplements, the state of affairs of supplementation may be mentioned in bankruptcy four. Some excessive protein meals resources are:

•Chicken

•Turkey

•Steak

•Protein powders

•Eggs

•Peanuts (or considered one of a type nut assets)

•Peanut butter (or distinctive kinds of nut butter)

•Chickpeas

The very last macronutrient is fats. Fat is regularly visible as a 'lousy' macronutrient, and a few humans think fat must be avoided altogether. However, fats isn't necessarily a awful factor. Fat can be broken down into 4 sections; trans fat, saturated fat, monounsaturated fat, and polyunsaturated fat. Trans and saturated fat are seen because the 'bad' fat, while monounsaturated and polyunsaturated fat are considered due to the fact the 'healthy' fats. The 'risky' fat are seemed for inflicting higher LDL, terrible levels of cholesterol, better LDL degrees are diagnosed for inflicting blood and coronary coronary heart deceases. 'Good' fats, however, are stated for doing the complete opposite, reducing LDL tiers and lowering the chances of coronary heart decease. Once yet again, the amount of fats you need to eat on a every day foundation depends to your dreams and modern-day body facts. Some 'well' fat property are:

•Fish

•Nuts

•Nut butters

•Avocados

Chapter 13: Supplementation

On to the situation of supplementation. People who're beginning their fitness journey frequently have the equal questions about supplements. The first question human beings typically have a tendency to invite is 'Are dietary supplements steroids?', and the answer is not any. Supplements contain natural substances which may be discovered in everyday meals belongings, even as steroids are artificial approaches of growing hormones.

The second question people often ask is 'Are dietary nutritional supplements important?' and all over again the answer isn't always any. As stated, supplements encompass the same vitamins regular meals does. Therefore you can devour the identical vitamins from eating regular food. However, dietary supplements do have blessings. The most commonplace advantage of taking dietary nutritional supplements which include whey protein is the truth that it is less complicated to gain your every day quantity of protein consumption. Since protein powders usually exist of 70+ percent of protein, there are little to no extra macronutrients concerned, on the equal time as peanuts, for instance, include a whole lot of fat. Next to that, the use of dietary dietary supplements collectively with whey protein will lower the prices consistent with gram of protein as compared to regular meals.

Up till now, whey protein has been the simplest stated complement. However, there are masses greater dietary dietary supplements, a number of a superb way to be explained.

Next to whey protein, there may be casein protein. Unlike whey protein, casein protein takes a long time to digest, because of this imparting your bloodstream with a regular release of amino acids lasting up to eight hours. Because of the enduring release, some of human beings eat casein protein proper in advance than they go to sleep, so their frame could be supplied with a normal amino acid launch at some degree in the night time time.

Another famous complement is BCAA's. BCAA stands for Branched-Chain Amino Acids. BCAA consists out of three critical amino acids: leucine, isoleucine and valine. These amino acids are the primary amino acids used for muscle constructing. BCAA's want for use in the path of, or straight away after your education. Because your body might now not need to digest the ones amino acids, they may be absorbed into your bloodstream manner quicker than some different protein shake. Therefore using BCAA nutritional nutritional supplements will substantially gain your muscle constructing manner.

Up till now, muscle building dietary nutritional supplements had been stated. However, there are various extra dietary nutritional supplements available. One of the arena's maximum famous workout supplements is pre exercise. Pre exercise is a supplement which incorporates various substances mixed to increase the blood float and rate the body with energy. In distinct phrases, pre exercising will you deliver a similarly enhance earlier than you begin your education so you can push your body to its limits. Pre exercise want to be taken 15 to 1/2 of-hour earlier than you begin your exercising. If you're a beginner inside the fitness and you want to start the use of pre-exercise, you need to start out with a lower dose, so your frame won't react inside the wrong way. Because pre wearing sports dietary supplements are supposed to offer you a boost, a few producers use factors banned by manner of using numerous true sports activities sports committees, so in case you want to use pre-workout, it's miles strongly counseled to check the materials.

The final supplement to be able to be cited is creatine. Creatine is every distinct complement which improves your performances within the gym. Creatine is a natural substance on your body. So what does creatine do? As cited, creatine improves your wellknown typical performance with the aid of assisting your body create energy. Thanks to the effects of creatine your body can bypass that 'more mile' and do the ones greater few reps. Of route, through being capable of do some greater reps, your improvement will growth as well. However, there are some awful effects while taking creatine. Firstly creatine is thought for water absorption this means that that your frame will store greater water than not unusual and therefore you will be lots much less likely to have lean-looking abs. Next to that, some humans argue that the use of creatine dietary dietary supplements motives balding, even though this has no longer formally been installation. The amount of creatine you need to use constant with day hasn't officially been set. However, maximum labels will show their preferred usage.

Chapter 14: Recovery and injuries

Muscles are not built inner of the gym. Even despite the fact that the manner of muscle increase starts offevolved inside the fitness center, the actual muscle boom takes area because of recuperation. By lifting weights you're developing tiny muscle tears, fiber is being broken. Because you push or pull sooner or later of a certain exercise, your muscle fibers are being lengthened therefore developing tiny tears in the fibers. Every muscle is hooked up to one or muscle bellies. To heal those muscle corporations your body upkeep or replaces the broken muscle fiber due to a cellular way associated with protein. This method includes protein synthesis in which your frame releases a first rate quantity of protein to repair broken muscle groups. The released protein, amino acids, will restore or update the damaged muscle fibers because of this developing extra muscle mass. Protein synthesis takes area each 48 hours. Therefore it's far endorsed to have at least 48 hours amongst education the equal muscle companies.

However, there are a few exceptions to this rule. Some muscle groups can be skilled two times indoors 48 hours. These muscle agencies are your abdominals (abs) and your calves.

The majority of your body's restoration takes place while you sleep. That's why it is vital to offer your body with the amount of relaxation it wishes. Preferably an man or woman need to sleep a mean 8 hours in keeping with day. However, a number of people aren't capable of get 8 hours of sleep in each and each day. Even notwithstanding the truth that eight hours of sleep is top-quality, 7 hours of sleep will despite the fact that offer your frame with enough rest.

Another remember to say is accidents. Whatever sport you workout, some thing exercising you do, there's constantly a hazard of having injured. You can do a few subjects to try to prevent injuries from occurring to a positive amount. Most of those strategies have already been referred to together with resting and the use of proper strategies. However, there are one-of-a-kind techniques to try to save you injuries together with stretching and foam rolling.

Foam rolling is a self-rub down method that want to be used proper after your training. The consequences of foam rolling are much like you will get by using way of getting a actual massage. So how does foam rolling art work? By foam rolling the educated muscle organizations, you're developing strain at the muscle's trigger factors. By doing this, you are releasing anxiety from the muscle companies while you are loosening the muscle as nicely.

However, you shouldn't just blindly foam roll every muscle group. Even even though foam rolling is an powerful technique for training maximum of your muscle companies, you have to in no manner use a foam curler in your lower all over again. Instead of the use of a foam roller for your lower yet again, you have to use a lacrosse ball.

Next, to foam rolling, you want to stretch. Some humans stretch in advance than their exercising and others stretch afterwards. Stretching earlier than your workout is sufficient to heat and loosen up the muscular tissues, stretching after your exercising will save you your muscular tissues from tightening up.

Even despite the fact that there are a couple of strategies to try to prevent accidents, it's although possible to get injured. Whenever you get injured, it's essential to offer your muscle tissue time to get better. Whether you take time without work from the fitness center, this is essential, or train across the injured muscle employer, you generally have to use the injured muscle as low as viable.

How you need to deal with injuries is based upon on the shape of damage you've got had been given. Treating an harm want to both be completed with cryotherapy (bloodless treatment) or thermotherapy (thermal treatment). Cryotherapy want for use on every muscle institution, besides the decrease lower again. Cryotherapy need to be finished inside seventy two hours after the ache starts offevolved offevolved. However, below some conditions you shouldn't use cryotherapy, those activities being touchy pores and skin and advanced diabetes given that advanced diabetes want to motive overusing cryotherapy. Cold/ice packs and frozen vegetables are the most generally used products for cryotherapy.

Thermotherapy, or warm remedy, want for use for accidents lasting longer than seventy hours and decrease once more pain. Just as with cryotherapy, thermotherapy want for use cautiously if a person has superior diabetes. Both cryotherapy and thermotherapy are commonly used strategies for treating brief-term accidents. When accidents keep over an prolonged period you ought to visit a licensed expert for in addition treatment.

Chapter 15: Mindset

So some distance the subjects have especially been approximately the physical detail of health and despite the fact that fitness about bodily fitness, your intellectual health and mind-set play a massive feature in staying on course. The cause maximum humans stop jogging out isn't due to a lack of time, it is now not because of fitness problems, however it's due to a loss of motivation. Both beginners and professional lifters despite the fact that conflict with actually attending to the gym. Once you are inside the gym, you can go through with a few thing exercise you had planned, however going to the gymnasium is the principle battle. There are a couple of strategies to make sure you hit the gym every single week. The first detail you could do is ready a ordinary date to transport exercising. Every week you will hit the health club the same day of the week round that equal time. After some time, it will become a addiction to go to the health club, and you could have fewer struggles attending to the gym. Another motivator is getting a exercising buddy. When you hit the gymnasium with a chum, you will enjoy obligated to go to the gym, and it's far going to be all of the greater amusing to have a friend proper at the side of you.

Some human beings create a praise machine. For instance, if a person goes to the fitness center times in step with week, they may be capable of eat that pizza at some degree inside the weekend. Or if they will exercise consultation within the morning, they'll have the night time off. Using reward systems just like the ones can be a incredible motivator to get to the fitness center. Of course, you shouldn't cross overboard and reward yourself with junk meals after each and every exercising. If you'll lose 4 hundred energy via aerobic and consume three hundred power nicely sincerely really worth of junk food after your exercising, you wasted the bulk of your exercising.

Next to having the motivation to go to the health club, it is a splendid issue to set goals.

When you location a fine purpose, you're greater stimulated to artwork within the course of that intention instead of simply going to the health club, doing some stuff and notice what happens. You may also have dreams you need to achieve inner a brief-time period, or you may have goals for the long term. Setting short-time period, as well as prolonged-time period goals, is a amazing manner of going after what you need. By dividing your lengthy-term intention into quick-term dreams, you may work inside the course of your ultimate purpose on the equal time as nevertheless conducting specific goals a great manner to offer you a boost in each yourself warranty and motivation. Another manner to provide you extra motivation to acquire your goals is through making your desires public. Tell your pals what your goals are or put up your goals on social media. Even although it is able to appear frightening to make your desires public, it's going to increase the probabilities of you accomplishing your goals for the purpose that you have now have been given humans counting on you.

Another detail that's related to placing your goals is retaining music of your progress. If you're on the lookout for to benefit strength, write down how masses your weights have improved or degree the elements of your frame you want to grow. If you're looking to lose fat, diploma your body fat percent on a regular foundation and weigh yourself. Weigh-ins have to be finished at a normal 2d, for say on every occasion after your final workout of the week or every Monday morning. The cause for that is the distinction for your body weight inside the direction of the day, for say, your body isn't inside the same kingdom whilst you wake up than it is inside the night time time. Keeping music of your development will offer you with an instance of ways powerful your health plan is and offer you with motivation every time you spot some improvement.

However, the scale doesn't say the whole thing. Even although weighing yourself is pretty of a hallmark how subjects are going, it does now not inform the whole tale. Weighing your self handiest display you the growth or lower in weight, however it might no longer say anything about your muscle groups or fat loss. For instance, a person looking to lose fats does now not always have to lose weight to reap their desires. If you go to the gymnasium with the intention of dropping weight by the use of doing every cardio and lifting you may enjoy an growth in muscular tissues as nicely, therefore you could even though lose fat at the identical time as not dropping any weight due to the increase is your muscular tissues. Therefore it's endorsed to degree your body fats and muscle groups further to weighing yourself.

Chapter 16: Tools

Previously, subjects which incorporates macronutrients, foam rolling and body fat measurements were referred to. For such and masses of different health subjects there are beneficial tools to help and manual you towards your dreams. In this economic catastrophe, some beneficial and clean fitness device might be mentioned.

The first device a awesome way to be defined is a calorie and macronutrient tracker called MyFitnessPal. MyFitnessPal is available in each the shape of a internet website and an app. Instead of getting to jot down down the entirety you consume and having to appearance up the amount of calories and macronutrients you may short look for a specific product or take a look at the barcode of the product. Because MyFitnessPal comes inside the form of a cell app you can use it everywhere you want and continues tune of something you devour at some stage in the day. When you sign on for MyFitnessPal, you can must supply your duration, body weight and your health cause and then MyFitnessPal will offer you with a encouraged amount of power and macronutrients.

However, there are higher processes of locating the proper amount of calories and macronutrients. There are numerous net web sites in which you can find a calorie/macronutrient recommendation primarily based totally on your age, gender, weight, duration and fitness desires. Of direction, seeing a dietist or virtually everyone with a qualification in making eating regimen plans might be capable of provide you with a customized estimate on the subject of macronutrients.

Even despite the fact that developing a diet plan is the first step, retaining music of your development is step two. As referred to in the preceding monetary break, using a frame fat measurement tool is a superb way of checking your improvement. There are a couple of techniques of checking your body fat measurements, of which the most accurate may be a DEXA take a look at, however DEXA scans are exceptionally costly and require seeing a professional. Therefore the most typically used method of measuring frame fats is with the useful resource of manner of the use of a frame fat calliper. Body fats callipers are smooth to apply and really cheaper. However, the accuracy of a frame fats calliper is doubtable, and it is able to not supply 100% accurate size.

Besides system regarding weight benefit or loss, there are specific equipment, which incorporates foam rollers and yoga mats. Foam rollers, as said in the preceding economic smash, are a less expensive manner of having the effects of massage through the usage of manner of using self-massage techniques. Foam rollers exist in plenty of shapes and forms and range from distinctly less pricey to pretty luxurious. Yoga mats are very useful as properly. Even despite the fact that yoga mats are mainly, due to the fact the call already suggests, used for yoga, they're also beneficial for stretching. Just like foam rollers, yoga mats exist in one-of-a-type sizes and additionally range in fee.

Next to machine to apply earlier than and after your exercising, there are distinctive device to use in some unspecified time in the future of your workout. One of these equipment is a weightlifting belt. Weightlifting belts are a stabiliser in your lower decrease back while lifting heavy weights on physical activities collectively with deadlifts, squats and overhead presses. As a beginner you received't need to apply a weightlifting belt due to the fact the quantity of weight you're lifting most probable received't be extra than your bodyweight. Some humans use lifting straps as nicely to have a higher grip at some stage in tremendous bodily video games, whereas different humans use lifting gloves.

Of course, there are numerous other equipment than the range as said above of system. However, surely as with supplementation, those gear are just system, they aren't vital to attain your goals. Even no matter the reality that a number of the ones device should make it simpler to gain your goals, it is although viable to go together with out them.

Chapter 17: Reach your dreams

In this ebook, numerous fitness topics were said. Hopefully, all the statistics and pointers can be beneficial in guiding your towards your dreams and desires. Of path, there may be manner extra data approximately health and fitness obtainable. There are loads upon loads of books, articles and films that assist you to achieve your desires and teach you about health and the fitness business enterprise. Whether your aim is to step on degree and do a health competition in the end, or in case you need to lose some pounds, there can be normally a way to obtain your dreams and push yourself similarly than you can ever consider. Don't be your personal roadblock by manner of pronouncing you can not do this otherwise you can not do that, you may. Millions of humans have been wherein you're, and thousands and hundreds have human beings have reached their goals.

What higher time to begin attaining your dreams than now? Every day you wait is any other day you may were getting within the route of your goals. Yes, there are numerous excuses to be made as to why you're now not capable of workout or consume healthily, but the fact of the hassle is, there can be continually a manner if you need it awful enough. Do you want to control your life or are you letting your existence manage you? Just think about how brilliant you may sense whilst you've misplaced those few pounds or when you've stepped on diploma and confirmed hundreds of human beings what improvement you've made.

By studying this ebook, you've got already set up which you want to make a danger on your existence. Now it's time a good manner to comply with up on it. Use the facts from this e book and start your health adventure in recent times.

Chapter 18: The Benefits of Physical Fitness

What is physical fitness? Why is it vital? What are you able to do to advantage it? The solutions to a majority of those questions can be addressed inside the chapters to observe. First, allow's begin with a easy definition of what being physically match clearly technique. Being physically in form has excellent meanings for one-of-a-kind humans. The international elegance marathoner's definition of health is a lot unique than in all likelihood that of a husband and a spouse looking to be a part of a fitness center for the primary time, or an important student taking element in a bodily schooling elegance. One issue is for positive, however: being bodily fit will permit us to perform all additives of each day life with out feeling worn out or fatigued. Being physical match moreover gives our our our our bodies the capability to combat off existence threatening illnesses which includes diabetes, most cancers and coronary heart disorder. Physical health is product of many components. All of those mechanisms permit us to execute our every day responsibilities with an entire lot tons much less try. These additives consist of cardiovascular fitness, flexibility, muscular strength and vitamins. These interlocking mechanisms represent the bodily in shape character. Shoveling snow, raking leaves and on foot to the store all end up an awful lot a lot much less tough for the physical suit character. Developing a smooth fitness plan that consists of all of these vital quantities will positioned us nicely on our way to a wholesome manner of existence and a extra effective life. An computerized, technological society has helped to create a sedentary way of life which in turn has generated the want for a whole fitness plan. The amazing part of it's miles that doesn't ought to be hard and it does now not want to consume all your time. You can pick out the activities and physical sports you need to perform and boom a plan that meets your character desires and pursuits. Now let us have a test the four training of health, and the manner each of them will permit you to acquire your private private dreams.

Cardiovascular Fitness

Cardiovascular health may be the maximum critical element of the physical healthful person. The term cardiovascular refers back to the coronary coronary coronary heart and its surrounding tissue. It is essential to recognize that the coronary heart is a muscle; like each extraordinary muscle in the body, in case you exercise it, you will decorate its average overall performance. The coronary coronary heart's task is to pump the blood during the body to all tissues and organs. Exercise and bodily interest can assist the coronary coronary coronary heart to do its mission extra correctly. Your coronary coronary heart can pass one in each of methods; beat faster to growth blood float, or beat slower with greater ordinary overall performance by the usage of the usage of sending extra blood with every beat. So as you probably decided out, a healthy man or woman is much more likely to have a lower beat regular with minute coronary heart price, in region of the no longer really worth person, whose coronary heart has to artwork a lot greater tough to accumulate the same blood waft. In the evaluation segment of "Health and Fitness for Beginners", you may discover ways to calculate your resting coronary heart fee in addition to your exercising coronary coronary heart fee that will help you decide and display your fitness degree. Think approximately this, a physically healthy individual may additionally moreover furthermore have a resting coronary coronary heart rate of 60 beats according to minute in place of an not worth individual whose resting coronary coronary heart rate can be 80 beats in line with minute. That's 20 beats a minute more over their entire life. Whose heart will placed on out faster?

Blood, veins and arteries are also large benefactors inside the our bodies of physical wholesome individuals. Since the blood, veins and arteries are vital for wearing all the critical vitamins inside the path of the body, you can see why you need to keep this tool wholesome. Fats are an vital nutrient for your our our bodies; however, in greater they can trigger the formation of ldl ldl cholesterol that might acquire to your arteries. These fatty deposits can shape on the partitions of your arteries in flip restricting essential blood go with the float. The illness due to this fats growth is known as atherosclerosis. It can turn out to be extremely risky while it blocks the artery and oxygen can not get to the coronary coronary heart, inflicting a coronary heart attack. Regular bodily exercise has been verified to enhance the efficiency of blood flow, and in lots of times, enhance the community of arteries and veins at some level inside the coronary coronary coronary heart and body. Another important evaluation is knowing and understanding your levels of cholesterol. We will speak greater approximately this inside the evaluation section of this e-book. All you need to apprehend proper now's that there is right ldl ldl ldl cholesterol (HDL) and awful cholesterol

(LDL). You need to hold that LDL range low (below a hundred) and that HDL range excessive (above 60). Needless to mention, physical hobby and exercise will try this for you.

Since the coronary coronary heart and lungs have to art work in conjunction together, the breathing device becomes essential in the fashionable cardiovascular health of an person. Your breathing machine is crafted from the throat and lungs and is accountable for bringing that oxygen from the air into your body. Oxygen, which enters the blood, offers those important nutrients that we mentioned earlier. The easy through- product comprised of this oxygen blood trade, carbon dioxide, is expelled from the frame as waste. The aggregate of the coronary heart and lungs allows to supply the essential nutrients to the frame at the equal time as ridding the body of wastes. Again, workout can beautify the overall overall performance of the lungs, which in turn, improves tiers of cardiovascular health.

Muscles and Nerves

Muscle cells are essential whilst performing any cardiovascular health workout because of the truth on the equal time as they're advanced, they allow your body to keep to transport over extended intervals of time without fatiguing. Nerves, as an alternative, reply to messages from the brain and assist with muscular contraction in components of the frame collectively with the arms and legs. During exercising, your mind communicates alongside facet your muscle companies to obtain precise designed responses. By looking at your motion inside the path of exercising, you emerge as greater privy to the mind-muscle interaction. You can now start to train your involved tool to perform in way that you want it to. Balance and posture can be superior as you are making yourselves consciously aware of this mind muscle connection throughout your exercising workouts. The nerves throughout the coronary coronary heart, on the other hand, function involuntarily; this is why the coronary coronary heart maintains to conquer with out the thoughts telling it to acquire this. Remember: if you may lower the coronary heart fee, you could improve the performance of your cardiovascular tool. You can enhance each of those structures with an high-quality fitness and exercising plan.

How an entire lot Physical Activity

The depth and length of physical interest will another time range from character to man or woman. You will want to decide how fit you want to come to be. You can even want to determine how a brilliant deal time each day you need to devote in your fitness plan. Many professionals agree that at least 20 minutes of fitness three-4 times each week will enhance the performance of the cardiovascular device. So, with that in mind, 20 mins turns into an tremendous place to begin for maximum beginners.

Cardiovascular Activities

There are many bodily sports activities, physical activities and sports that train the cardiovascular gadget. Team sports sports along facet soccer and basketball offer notable exercises and help to beautify the cardiovascular system. For those of you that pick out man or woman sports activities, dance, walking, cycling, swimming and aerobics provide alternatives to enhance your fitness. That is the splendor of physical health; "vintage faculty workout" does now not have to be the concept of your schooling. You can pick out the sports you experience the most to help you decorate your preferred fitness level.

Flexibility

Flexibility is defined because the functionality to move your muscle tissues and joints through a complete form of motion. It is that one element of health that most people spend the least quantity of time on, or they determined on to do no longer some thing the least bit. Working on correct flexibility takes time, so for plenty human beings it's miles the maximum tedious part of the workout plan. We comprehend, however, that being bendy has many fitness benefits. By stretching your muscle organizations on a everyday basis, you can assist prevent harm and decrease muscle pain. Flexibility allows with yet again fitness and improves our posture. Flexibility can help you in everyday each day existence competencies which incorporates painting and raking. Flexibility can decorate athletic overall performance consisting of developing a backswing in tennis and golfing. For runners, growing flexibility manner growing your stride period, which in turn, manner covering extra ground inside the identical amount of time. So, as you could see flexibility will serve an important characteristic in a health plan.

Muscular Strength

When we recollect power education, the vision of frame builders in a sweaty, overcrowded weight room entails thoughts.

Those days are prolonged lengthy long long gone. Sure, in case you want to trying to find out this kind of gym you may discover it, however this isn't what the bulk people need to certainly beautify our muscular health. There are many alternatives available even as seeking out a way to improve your energy. Clubs, health facilities home gyms in addition to frame weight bodily activities are only some of the options which may be now to be had to you. No one desires to be intimidated whilst project a strength schooling software program. There are alternatives for clearly all people. After analyzing "Health and Fitness for Beginners" you may all have the enough records to with a piece of luck stroll into any fitness center and understand precisely what you're doing.

So, what are the advantages of being more potent? Improved self-image, better everyday fitness and stepped forward common overall performance on each day duties are all blessings of stepped forward strength profits. Strength training at the same time as finished on a everyday foundation will hold healthful blood strain tiers similarly to lower levels of cholesterol inside the blood. Your bones become stronger and as a give up stop result lower your chance of osteoporosis, a disease that weakens the bones. Like flexibility, muscle power decreases harm and additionally allows you get over injuries quicker. Again, there is probably many alternatives on the same time as selecting a energy education application. Machine fashion schooling as visible in health golf equipment can be very famous; free weights and dumbbells are every different technique; and body weight bodily activities are quality for humans truly getting started out out. You can select the method that first-rate suits your desires.

Nutrition

What you located into your frame serves because of the reality the gas to help you entire the obligations critical to get thru life on a each day foundation. The query is what's the vital gas favored that allows you to assist whole those each day obligations? The way to that question is not an clean one. People are available all particular sizes, a long term and weights; a few are greater lively, at the same time as others lead sedentary lives. The United States Department of Agriculture's food pyramid has served as the idea for all Americans at the way you need to eat every and each day. Although this model has been round for decades, it nevertheless maintains to alternate and evolve. One component is for superb, however: your body desires nutrients to help you grow and live on. Our frame goals nutrients from six important organizations. These groups include: carbohydrates, fats, proteins, nutrients, minerals and of path water. Carbs, fat and proteins provide the energy had to make it thru each day. The probabilities of each fed on will variety primarily based on the characteristics indexed above. The contemporary-day "My Plate" pointers from the USDA embody picks from proteins, greens, culmination, grains and dairy.

Vegetables and grains make up the largest portions in the USDA's guidelines. Carbohydrates provide us with our maximum vital supply of electricity. There are number one varieties of carbohydrates: smooth and complicated. Complex carbohydrate sugars are observed in such food as complete grain breads, cereals and veggies. The nutrients in the ones carbs, which is probably more "dense," are more useful to us. Simple carbs along side the ones determined in candy, cake and soda encompass extra energy, however moreover include fewer vital vitamins and minerals. Fiber is likewise a complicated carbohydrate; it's far a totally important nutrient in a wholesome diet plan. Foods which includes uncooked greens, cereals and nuts offer fibers critical each day. Proteins are the nutrients that hold, construct and restore your frame cells. Proteins are located in animal products together with milk, eggs, fish and meat. Proteins moreover offer you with electricity, and on the same time, include fewer power than carbohydrates and fat. Fats alternatively are critical for the boom and restore of cells; they dissolve sure vitamins and delivery them to our cells. Fats are labeled as each saturated or non-saturated. Unsaturated fat come from such additives as fish, nuts and olives to name a few. Saturated fat come from meals collectively with milk, butter and meat. Saturated fats along thing trans fats (similar to the ones placed in margarine) have long been concept to be a purpose of ldl cholesterol buildup in our arteries and a contributing component inside the improvement of atherosclerosis. The contemporary studies now show that saturated fats together with the ones determined in eggs aren't as terrible for you as as soon as believed. The USDA even though recommends that saturated fat make up no more than 10 % of your healthy dietweight-reduction plan. Vitamins, minerals and water are all essential vitamins and play a vital position in keeping us all wholesome.

Chapter 19: Assess Your health

In financial ruin 1, you found that it is no huge mystery that fitness and exercising offer you with many benefits. To create your fitness utility and head ahead to your journey to advantage those advantages, you need to first take a look at your modern stage of fitness. In this monetary ruin, we're able to address several forms of clinical and bodily fitness assessments. These assessments are designed to help you get an concept of in that you're now and in that you need to transport in relation to border composition and cardiac health. Most of these self-assessments can be finished by means of using easy circle of relatives gadgets or lots less steeply-priced health assessment charts and gear. We will use a few simple sports activities that will help you look into your present day bodily fitness associated reputation. This in flip will help you whilst you start to layout your personal character workout. We can also even check some easy to do frame composition checks an splendid way to provide you with instantaneous comments as it relates for your final body composition desires. Finally, we will display you a few smooth exams that may be administered at home on the manner to offer you a few heaps wanted facts in regards in your contemporary-day fitness reputation. Many of the exams and tests that we're capable of percent on this financial disaster require some degree of physical readiness. It is usually an first rate idea to look a medical doctor earlier than starting any exercise software program. Although the exams are not physical grueling, they may purpose pain to a few oldsters which are new to fitness or have never undertaken an workout software inside the past.

Physical Exercise Self-Assessment

To get commenced out in any workout utility you need to first offer you with an area to begin. In order to installation this location to start you have to find out in which your current-day health level lies. This start line will be exquisite for every body, and is probably based totally definitely to your revel in, way of existence and expertise. Millions of younger Americans take part in bodily training in our faculties. Many of them are examined on their health degrees with the beneficial resource of taking part each three hundred and sixty five days in a nation, community or countrywide fitness checking out application. These exams offer pertinent facts to their directors on how properly our younger people are conditioned, and the manner they stack up with one-of-a-type more youthful humans nationally and round the world. The physical checks that we are able to introduce to you're very comparable; however, they'll be designed to house all levels of fitness. Therefore, it's far critical to see a medical doctor to decide if your frame is ready to perform those easy health tests. Remember to start off slowly and to prevent even as the carrying sports grow to be too tough or painful. If you can not complete one of the checks that's adequate; you may normally regulate them or make adjustments on your very last fitness prescription. Establishing your beginning fitness diploma will allow you to inspect your private non-public desires as properly assist you to benefit powerful manipulate of your complete fitness and well being. The health checking out gadgets may be divided into three categories: 1. Cardiovascular 2. Strength and three. Flexibility. The results from the ones exams will assist to determine your regions of energy and what your goals for improvement could be. These consequences may additionally provide you with instantaneous comments and could lay the foundation for your very very own non-public bodily health plan. Let's check the checks. Remember to document your results on a chunk of paper. We will examine the information later.

Strength

1. Modified take a seat down- ups: This check is done lying to your lower back on a mild ground together with a carpet or mat when you have one to be had. Your knees want to be bent among ninety and 100

twenty ranges. Your ft need to be slightly aside and your toes want to be flat at the ground. Fold your fingers all through your chest. One sit down-up is recorded on every occasion you touch as a minimum one elbow in your thigh. Return on your starting role for your lower back and maintain. You have one minute to complete as many changed take a seat-the united states you could. If you haven't executed take a seat-usain a while otherwise you become worn-out or out of breath, you can want to stop early. Your rating might be the wide variety of correct changed take a seat down-americayou executed inside the one minute length.

2. Push-ups: This take a look at is finished mendacity face down on a tender ground. Your hands have to be positioned shoulder width apart. You have to be up to your toes alongside side your legs some inches aside. Now, push up till your hands are instantly and your head, again and legs are in a right away line. Lower your frame until your elbows attain ninety degrees on the equal time your

decrease lower again need to stay in a immediately line. Each time you come up you get credit score for one push up. Unlike the sit-up take a look at, you can carry out as many push-america you can till you have a shape breakdown. It is terrific to have a accomplice watch you to ensure you carry out the frenzy-u.S. Of americanicely. If you have got were given by no means completed push-ups, or have no longer completed them in some time, you may need to stop once they begin to end up too hard. Your rating can be calculated via the range of push- usayou carried out in advance than breaking form or rhythm.

Cardiovascular

three.   One—mile Walk/Run/Jog: For this hobby, you can need to go to a jogging song or the very least have a one-mile path laid out somewhere near your own home. Most taking walks tracks are four laps to the mile. In this check, your score is probably based totally totally on the quantity of time it takes you to finish the only-mile direction. You will want a forestall watch to diploma some time. You might also walk, run or jog or a aggregate of the 3 to finish your one-mile. Your score may be based totally certainly at the time to finish the mile route. If this hobby turns into tough, undergo in thoughts you could walk to finish the mission. Write down some time whilst you finish.

Flexibility

4.   Hamstring Stretch: For this check, you'll want a ruler or yardstick. Sit down on a flat floor along side your ft just a few inches aside. Place the start of the ruler or outside stick at a point included up with the returned of your heels. Lean in advance and attain with the arms together as far over the ruler as you could for three repetitions. On the zero.33 repetition, try to hold the location over the ruler for so long as you could on the equal time as a associate measures what number of inches past your feet that you have extended.

Your score should be measured to the closest inch.

Health Related Testing

Resting Heart Rate

The extensive shape of instances your coronary heart beats in one minute may be a identifying problem of your contemporary health degree. Generally, maximum medical medical doctors agree that a regular resting coronary heart rate tiers from 60-a hundred beats consistent with minute; however, there are numerous elements that would alter the variety of your coronary coronary heart price within the path of a ordinary day. Too a first-rate deal caffeine, smoking, sure medicines, and strain are all elements that may exchange your heart price during a regular day. Many human beings may additionally additionally sincerely occur to be born with a immoderate heart rate at the same time as others may be born with a far decrease one. One element is for high-quality, but: the coronary heart is a muscle which may be conditioned and modified. Most well-conditioned athletes will find themselves within the decrease kind of ordinary coronary coronary heart fee whilst an unconditioned character will show off a higher pulse price. An rather immoderate or low coronary coronary heart charge can be a pre-cursor of an underlying hassle. Needless to say, that is a few detail you must take a look at out in conjunction with your clinical physician.

Ok, permit's get started out out out on checking your private individual coronary coronary heart charge. For this test you will want a stop watch and a accomplice. There are locations you could resultseasily test to get an accurate coronary coronary heart charge or pulse price. One technique is to location your first and second arms gently on the carotid artery, placed on the neck on the element of the windpipe. The second method is to diploma the coronary heart beat on the wrist. Simply region fingers lightly at the thumb element of your wrist. Either of those places may be excellent, and actually checking your pulse rate from each locations is even better. You will perform this take a look at times for higher accuracy using one or every of the techniques formerly said. Sit down in a chair or on the ground and place your palms on your preferred place. Next, have your associate take keep of a save you watch or timer and clock one minute at the same time as you rely the amount of beats. Record your rating for trial one and do it a second time to test for accuracy. If you're within some beats on the second trial this is exceptional. If you're way off, you could want to begin the test over and do not forget checking the heart beat in a completely unique location.

Now that you have your rating, you could see in which you healthy inner that 60-one hundred variety. This score will function a future reference of fitness as you development through your workout programs. As we said earlier than, the coronary coronary heart is a muscle that can be modified and conditioned. If your coronary heart beats at a lower fee, it is running extra effectively and does now not want to artwork as hard to pump all the blood inside the route of your frame. Your aim need to be to lower your resting coronary coronary heart price as you improvement through your health utility.

Maximum Heart Rate

Before you get began to your workout plan, it is crucial to decide how hard you must art work your coronary heart in some unspecified time in the future of every exercise consultation. In different phrases, what number of beats in step with minute is the edge in your non-public workout. Many formulation were designed to help you determine what the most variety of coronary coronary heart beats want to be at some stage in one minute of workout. The vintage college method of taking the extensive variety 220 and subtracting your age has end up the most as an alternative used method of figuring out maximum coronary coronary coronary heart charge (MHR). Many opponents of this system declare that it fails to recall own family heritage further to such things as contemporary fitness degree and top and weight. The additives additionally assumes that anybody have the same resting heart fee at a given age, and that our MHR price declines at the identical diploma for every person. As a result this technique should variety as many as 20-30 beats in step with minute. Another approach includes subtracting zero.7 X age from 208. In my case, it makes a distinction of five beats normal with minute at the upside. The maximum correct degree can be to visit your nearest biomechanical laboratory and feature the scientific doctors discern that out for you. Unfortunately, that is way too impractical and sincerely expensive. So permit's stay with one of the antique university formula to determine our MHR. Even no matter the reality that it is able to be off through the usage of a few beats this will offer us a beginning issue and feature a splendid manual. Your purpose for the duration of workout can be in no way to transport over the range which you derive from your components of preference. Target Exercise Heart Rate

To gauge your intensity all through your workout, you want to determine at what degree to artwork the coronary coronary coronary heart within the course of exercising. This degree is called your Target Exercise Heart Rate. To determine your Target Exercise Heart Rate, you want to first decide at what degree of intensity you will be education. For those of you actually starting, or who absolutely want to perform at a slight level of depth, you'll use a components of 50%- 60% of your most coronary coronary coronary heart fee in which you simply calculated above. For the ones looking for to pursue a more active diploma of exercising, you will use 70%-eighty% of your maximum coronary coronary heart rate. Now get out your calculators and decide out your purpose coronary coronary coronary heart charge region. Moderate exercisers will multiply .Five or .6 X MHR. Vigorous or extra excessive exercisers will multiply .7 or .8 X MHR.

Whatever range you derive from this components becomes your baseline for your aim exercising region. Your MHR serves as the brink of your purpose workout place. Using a forty 365 days vintage for instance and going with the antique university gadget of 220-age, 100 and eighty may end up the MHR for this man or woman. Assuming a mild degree of exercise at 60%, we might then multiply 0.6 X 100 80 and offer you with a baseline vicinity extensive type of 108. To advantage a training impact this forty three hundred and sixty five days vintage ought to need to exercise amongst 108-one hundred 80 beats consistent with minute throughout the complete exercise. If you want to check to look if you are in the intention coronary heart price region, actually save you your exercising for a short 2d and take a look at your pulse for 10 seconds. Next, multiply this big variety with the useful resource of way of 6 to check your cutting-edge coronary coronary coronary heart price. Note how lots "wiggle room" you have got interior your intention coronary coronary coronary heart price sector.

Exercise Recovery Rate

The amount of time it takes after exercise to get decrease returned on your resting coronary coronary coronary heart fee is known as the exercise restoration fee. Complete restoration after exercise relies upon on many elements. It depends at the depth of your exercise, further to how close you got here in your most coronary coronary coronary heart charge. It additionally depends to your contemporary health stage. A individual this is in brilliant form receives higher lots faster than someone who isn't always. Another manner to expose that is to test your coronary coronary heart rate at once after exercising. Check your carotid artery, counting the beats for thirty seconds. Once you get this amount multiply with the useful resource of way of to get your workout coronary heart rate. Now wait for 2 mins and test your carotid pulse another time. Most health workers agree a drop of 15-20 beats is considered everyday, a drop of 12 beats or an awful lot much less is a sign of horrible fitness or perhaps even some early cardiovascular caution symptoms and signs and symptoms and symptoms. Needless to say strolling out on a everyday basis can help on your workout recuperation rate.

Body Composition Assessments

Body Mass Index (BMI)

BMI is a nationally recognized assessment of standard body fats. The check measures popular body fats primarily based totally on a gadget that calculates a person's weight because it pertains to their top. BMI can function a amazing indicator of an man or woman's weight problems and the apparent fitness risks that go along with being obese. Diseases which encompass stroke, coronary heart disease, immoderate blood pressure and excessive cholesterol are all related to immoderate BMI's. It is crucial to phrase that BMI is nice one such tool that may be used to assess health, and that it could now not be suitable for definitely each person. Shorter, more muscular people may additionally fall into the overweight class despite the fact that they may be in terrific form and encompass little or no frame fats. Similarly, an out of form skinny person may additionally furthermore score inside the ordinary class for BMI despite the fact that she or he famous little or no muscular tissues, and a immoderate percent of body fats. BMI is merely a trademark and device to assess obesity in an individual. To decide a score on your personal BMI you may use the chart below or considered simply one of most of the calculators which might be furnished on line. A BMI score of 18.Five-24.Nine places a person inside the regular magnificence for weight and peak. A rating at 25 and above categorizes someone within the obese through obese categories for BMI.

00003.Jpeg

Skin fold Measurement

A better way to decide body fats percent consists of skinfold calipers. In your BMI length, top and weight measurements did no longer endure in thoughts variations in body fats in comparison with lean frame mass. Skinfold calipers may be able to do that. The skinfold device measures frame fats with the useful resource of manner of the use of folds of pinched skin from across the body to provide a greater correct reading of frame fats percent. Skinfold calipers may be offered at maximum fitness and health shops, and additionally on Amazon for spherical ten to thirty dollars.

00004.Jpeg

Key places at the body for those measurements are on the waist, below the shoulder blade, the triceps and the quadriceps. You truely pinch the pores and pores and skin within the ones four regions pulling the fat far from the muscle and measuring the pinched pores and pores and skin together collectively with your calipers. The length may be in millimeters and it's far quality to take severa readings and use the common. For women, you could use the waist size (iliac crest) and the triceps measurement. For the grownup adult males you can use the thigh (quadriceps) and below the shoulder blade (subscapular). This is probably the only method to apply because it handiest calls for two readings. You then plug in those numbers into the Sloan equation for guys, Body Density=1.043-(zero.001327 x thigh skinfold in mm)-(0.00131x subscapular skinfold in mm). For ladies the technique is Body Density = 1.0764- (zero.0008 x iliac crest skinfold in mm)- (zero.00088 x triceps skinfold in mm). Acceptable frame fat opportunities for the overall population are in the 12-21% variety for men and inside the 17-28% variety for ladies. Keep in mind there are numerous unique tables, charts and method, and there are as tons as seven taken into consideration one among a kind locations in which to degree skinfolds. The Sloan technique appears to be the very first-rate approach to apply; but, a easy Google are seeking will provide you with many one of a kind techniques to interpret your skinfold length consequences.

Medical Self-Monitoring

Blood Pressure

During an annual bodily exam, the medical doctor frequently will administer a blood strain examination. During this examination, a cuff with a gauge or sphygmomanometer is located round your better arm. The cuff is pumped with air decreasing off circulate in your arm. The cuff is then slowly loosened because the scientific medical doctor makes use of a stethoscope to show your heart rate. The first reading the scientific physician will test due to the fact the cuff is loosened is your systolic stress. The second analyzing is your diastolic strain. Simply positioned, your systolic pressure (first range) measures the strain in your blood vessels while the coronary heart beats. The 2d substantial variety or diastolic stress measures the stress on your vessels even as the heart is at rest. A regular systolic variety is considered to be 100 and twenty or plenty less. A hundred and twenty-139 indicates pre-high blood stress and one hundred forty or over is excessive blood strain or excessive blood strain. A regular diastolic variety is 80 or much less. Pre-excessive blood stress is numerous amongst eighty-89 and excessive blood stress or excessive blood strain is a variety of 90 or better. High blood pressure or excessive blood strain is taken into consideration a chance issue for coronary coronary heart ailment and stroke. As you likely guessed, normal bodily interest and workout can decrease your blood stress into the ordinary variety or can help hold you from getting excessive blood strain. The extraordinary element approximately this check is which you no longer should wait one year for your physical to get your blood stress taken. You can purchase an much less luxurious package deal deal, or you could definitely go to your nearest drugstore and use their blood pressure monitoring machines.

Cholesterol

A ldl ldl cholesterol check is likewise one of these critical assessments that you want to get each 365 days at some point of your physical examination. This critical check will decide the danger that you are at for the buildup of plaque in your arteries. As all of us understand, this buildup can narrow the openings in our blood vessels inflicting atherosclerosis. Atherosclerosis is a pre cursor for plenty sorts of heart disease. To measure ldl ldl ldl cholesterol amount(s), the health practitioner will use a pattern of your blood to decide your preferred ldl ldl cholesterol quantity. A famous range below hundred mg/dl is considered appropriate on the equal time as pretty numerous over two hundred as lots as 239 mg/dl is considered borderline immoderate and any variety 240 and above is excessive. The physician may additionally moreover even offer you with numbers for the 2 lipoproteins that deliver the cholesterol thru your bloodstream. These lipoproteins are known as LDL (or horrible ldl cholesterol) and HDL (or proper ldl cholesterol). LDL is considered horrible because it clogs the arteries with plaque. HDL then again is considered appropriate as it receives rid of LDL ldl cholesterol from our arteries. An LDL wide variety under one hundred mg/dl is taken into consideration maximum essential, while some of above a hundred and sixty mg/dl is taken into consideration immoderate. For HDL ldl ldl ldl cholesterol pretty various beneath 50 is considered low for women, and below 40 is low for guys. An HDL amount above 60 mg/dl is taken into consideration to be notable. Once over again, regular bodily interest and workout can lessen the LDLs to your bloodstream, and at the identical time, boom your HDL's. Home take a look at kits for checking ldl ldl cholesterol are available however may be very costly. Make certain your stages are checked via a scientific doctor yearly, specifically when you have a circle of relatives records of coronary coronary heart disorder.

Chapter 20: The Elements of a Workout

As you put together to layout a fitness technique that suits your person dreams and goals, it's far important to understand the five crucial factors that want to be included right into a nicely-rounded fitness plan. These five elements want for use to help prepare your our our bodies to workout as well as hold you harm free. Make tremendous to combine the important time on your training so that it consists of all five of those vital elements. In this financial disaster, we can observe all five factors and the motives why they are critical in the improvement of genuine workout conduct. In the subsequent chapters, we're capable of delve more carefully into the sports and physical sports that want to be protected in each element.

Warming the Muscles

It might be very important to prepare the muscle mass on your our bodies just so they work effectively preceding to exercise. Similar to the way in that you warmness up your automobile in bloodless weather, your frame additionally want to be prepared to transport. Warm muscle tissues fireside extra efficiently during workout. Since the coronary heart is one of the most critical muscle tissues in your body, particular interest desires to be paid that it's miles warmed up properly. A amazing sluggish jog or a brisk stroll is a extremely good manner to elevate your coronary coronary heart price, and at the same time boost your popular frame temperature as a exquisite deal because the necessities essential for bodily interest. Five minutes is lots of time to heat the muscle tissue and get the coronary heart geared up for exercise. It is a fantastic idea to preserve your sweat pants and jackets on in some unspecified time in the future of this phase to preserve the muscle corporations warmth. This regular is a essential requirement for the reason that a heat muscle stretches extra with out issues and "fires" faster than a cold one. Let's get prepared to stretch.

Dynamic Stretching

A superb, dynamic stretching habitual accomplishes numerous things for you as you get geared up to begin your workout. It relaxes, loosens and elongates the muscle mass in coaching for physical hobby. A properly stretching software prevents accidents which incorporates pulled and strained muscular tissues. The flexibility this is obtained can also boom your stride duration, which in flip can ultimately growth your walking velocity. Dynamic stretching is the contemporary gold famous in the way people and organizations warmth up in coaching of exercising. These stretching exercises commonly require a good deal a good deal much less time than the antique static physical games that once ruled our "vintage university" hobby practices. Static stretching includes shielding the muscle in elongated positions for extended durations of time; somewhere amongst 30 seconds up to a minute or extra. Dynamic stretching, but: includes active stretching movements as you development over a completely unique distance; it is been demonstrated to be a more effective warm up for speed, agility and staying electricity type physical activities. It also can be completed in a much faster, more green quantity of time in evaluation to static stretching. Static stretching although has its place for your physical video games, however we trust it is time better spent on the notion of the hobby phase. Another plus to dynamic stretching is the capability to format the stretching habitual in accordance alongside facet your favored interest or exercise. In Chapter four, we're capable of study dynamic stretching carrying occasions and the manner to put in force them into your fitness programs.

Activity Phase

The interest section is wherein you may pick out the exercising packages, energy schooling programs and or the sport/hobby that you may be taking part in on any given day. This is where you may have the liberty to layout the personal application you want to take part in. This segment can embody such sports sports as cycling, swimming, on foot or weightlifting. It is actually as plenty as you, however recall it need to be an hobby that elevates your coronary heart rate into your non-public non-public intention exercise location. The splendor of your health plan is that it could be altered on a every day foundation, and may encompass as many one-of-a-kind activities as you preference. You may additionally discover that it could be smart to encompass power training into your workout each other day on the manner to balance your interest with other exercising orientated workout physical games. Most of the activities you chose can be divided up into this form of 3 education: cardio schooling, anaerobic education and strength schooling.

Aerobic Training

The time period cardio refers to the usage of oxygen. Aerobic activities are generally executed over prolonged periods of time; oxygen is provided to the muscle groups as needed. Such sports sports as distance walking, bike the usage of and pass u . S . A . Skiing are great examples of aerobic exercising. Aerobic sports, at the same time as done well over extended time, burn fats and serves as fantastic coronary coronary heart healthful cardiovascular workout.

Anaerobic Training

Anaerobic education entails quick, quick bursts of electricity which do no longer permit the coronary heart to deliver the crucial quantity of oxygen to the muscle tissue. That is why after participating in anaerobic education, your muscle groups now and again enjoy heavy or grow to be stiff, and lactic acid builds up within the muscle groups. Sprinting, energy lifting, and lengthy leaping are remarkable examples of anaerobic sports. Anaerobic sports activities are extra inclined to burn carbohydrates as their number one strength supply.

Strength Training

Strength schooling consists of the usage of unfastened weights, machines or frame weight physical video video games to beautify your muscular fitness. To grow to be more potent, you have to work your muscle groups more difficult than they may be generally familiar with art work. When you keep on with a regimented energy schooling application, your muscle corporations turn out to be extra efficient of their skills to carry out regular responsibilities. Raking leaves, shoveling snow and wearing groceries all come to be less complex while you are more potent. When designing a electricity training software program that fits your goals, you have to have a study many factors. Do you want to construct natural muscle strength or do you need to build muscular persistence? Do you want to elevate free weights, use machines or truly use your very private our our bodies to deliver the resistance? How lots time are you willing to spend each week on strength education? These are most of the questions you can must solution as you begin to layout your health plans.

Cool Down Phase

Just as it's far crucial to warmth the frame up in guidance for exercising, it is similarly critical to kick back the frame down after exercise. It is especially crucial if you just completed a strenuous cardio or electricity schooling workout. During a aerobic exercise along side strolling, your coronary coronary heart rate is nicely above your resting price, with any luck somewhere internal your goal location. As you complete your exercising, you need to slow the frame down and start your gradual descent into your resting coronary heart charge, and on the identical time, supply your frame temperature back off. After a electricity workout, your muscle groups grow to be worn-out and had been broken down. This cool down segment turns into critical to help muscle and tissue restore in addition to wellknown frame restoration. Going out for a slow clean jog or 5 mins on a treadmill at a slow tempo lets in the body to lighten up well.

Static Stretching

Once the chill out phase is completed, it now will become the proper time to put into impact a static stretching ordinary. Your muscles are tired, sore and consist of a waste product referred to as lactic acid. A first-class prolonged static stretching software program will beneficial beneficial resource in muscle restoration, and furthermore beneficial useful useful resource in the elimination of lactic acid. Static stretching can also even help you to growth your flexibility which turns into critical to the prevention of harm. Another bonus is that an growth in flexibility will boom your stride period, which in turn, may want to make you faster. You will research greater approximately static stretching within the subsequent monetary damage.

Monitor Your Fitness

Ideally you need to show your coronary heart price continually, in particular during the hobby phase and the restoration levels of your sporting activities. Having a save you watch on hand or wrist watch with a timer is extraordinarily critical. In bankruptcy 2, you located out tremendous techniques on how to test your resting, goal and recuperation coronary coronary coronary heart expenses. It is a good idea to check these readings throughout the improvement of your workout routines. This way you could see in case you are efficiently training on your specific schooling sector. Carry a logbook so that it will chart coronary coronary heart charge readings. These readings will help you find out how rapid your coronary coronary heart rate recovers after exercise, in addition to ensuring you're staying for your non-public exercise training zone.

Chapter 21: Flexibility

Many freshmen to health underestimate the significance of flexibleness because it pertains to their everyday fitness and health. As a keep in mind amount of fact, many beginners in truth leave this important element out of their exercise programs or spend little or no time on it. Whether you're greater youthful or old, flexibility has many health-associated blessings. In older adults hamstring (back of legs) flexibility can assist prevent decrease once more pain. In runners, calf and reduce ankle flexibility prevents an harm called shin splints. Making your muscular tissues extra bendy might also even improve your everyday posture. For athletes, it could assist to save you harm as nicely enhance your stride duration for on foot. Your golfing and tennis swings can emerge as longer and extra effective. Flexibility moreover aids in muscle recovery after workout. With all of those delivered blessings, why is it the hobby we devote the least quantity of time to?

In this economic disaster, we are capable of look at dynamic and static stretching. We will gift all of the stretching sporting activities available, and help you pick out the ones with the intention to advantage you maximum in your very personal personalized exercising plans. You can pick out out to do an ordinary flexibility plan, or a more specific plan geared to a selected exercising interest. As we present the sporting events, we're able to additionally percent the names of the muscle groups you may be stretching. It isn't always handiest crucial to understand the names of the muscle businesses, however it's miles in addition important to apprehend why you are stretching those muscle tissues. You will use the dynamic muscle bodily video games at the begin of your exercises, and use the static stretches throughout your sit back out phase on the belief of your exercising workouts.

Dynamic Stretching

Dynamic stretching is a exquisite manner to heat up for any health pastime. It is likewise a extraordinary manner to heat up for any organization or man or woman sports workout. Dynamic stretching is a extra prepared and a more efficient way to elevate the coronary coronary heart price. The purpose of dynamic stretching is to get the blood flowing and the body warmed up on the same time you are actively stretching all of the number one muscle groups. Time is used greater successfully even as you bear in mind that you could warmness up numerous fantastic muscle businesses on the identical time. This warmness up habitual entails transferring your body through a whole form of motion, at the same time as at the same time growing your blood waft. Dynamic stretching ought to be achieved slowly and grade by grade thru a completely unique distance of spherical ten to 20 yards. At no time need to you bounce, but on the same time you do not want to hold the stretch for too prolonged. You in reality want to set off and elongate the muscle after which hold to transport via the specified distance. As you go together with the go with the flow through the route, hold to lengthen the muscle, growing the period a bit more with every repetition. When dynamic stretching is finished successfully, you ought to revel in a gentle stretch in every precise muscle; on the equal time, elevating the coronary coronary heart charge in guidance for hobby.

Dynamic Stretching Routine

In order to prepare to your dynamic stretching recurring, it is a first-rate idea to map out a distance of about 10-20 yards counting on the distance you've got got to be had. All of the wearing events is probably carried out up and back thru this 10-20 backyard direction. Each motion must be well completed with accurate posture and shape. A mild stretch ought to be felt in the muscle you are activating. Keep your head up, and again at once each time feasible. Be careful now not to bounce and flow into slowly thru every workout. Remember in advance than you stretch, you want to warmness the muscle agencies in training for the stretch. A sluggish five minute heat up jog will suffice. Here are the dynamic stretching carrying activities:

1.   Thigh or Quadriceps Stretch- Begin to transport forward after which prevent and capture your proper ankle collectively together with your proper hand. Slowly pull the ankle and knee within the lower back of you as you maintain nicely posture. Stretch ought to be felt within the the the front of your leg or quad muscle. Move ahead and repeat with left leg. Continue to stretch alternating right and left quadriceps within the direction of the favored distance.

2.   Hamstring Stretch- The hamstring is the massive muscle in the lower returned of your leg. Move ahead as you lean your chest in advance over your right knee. Keep your leg right away as you factor your right toe up. You need to feel the stretch inside the once more of your leg. Repeat the moves as you bypass down the route with the left leg.

3.   Gluteal Stretch- Pull your proper knee for your chest with each fingers. Stretch need to be felt inside the gluteal muscle in other phrases your butt. As you float beforehand repeat this movement collectively with your left knee. A version and a extraordinary mindset of stretch may be attained by slowly pulling your knee greater towards the midline of your frame.

4.   Lunges- The lunge includes severa muscle organizations. When it's miles finished well, you'll experience a stretch inside the hips, glutes, hamstrings and quads. Keep your head up and again immediately as you lunge in advance and slowly press proper knee within the route of the floor; on the same time, growth the proper foot. Repeat the drill at the left trouble as you preserve via the direction.

5.   Calf Muscle/ Heel Walk- As you stroll ahead push off your heel and roll up onto your right toe. Continue to stroll and repeat collectively together with your left foot.

6. Groin Stretch- Move ahead as you raise proper knee and rotate it away and out of doors your body. Continue to transport ahead and repeat along side your left leg.

7. Hamstring Leg Kicks- Move beforehand as you slowly kick right foot upward in the direction of your right hand. Repeat with the left foot. This stretch again ought to be felt within the decrease back of the leg. Be careful not to kick too hard.

8. Lunge with a Twist- This exercising is much like the lunge besides that every time you lunge, twist and turn your waist. Lunge with the left foot and twist to the left facet. Repeat the motion at the proper component. The stretch should be felt within the hips, glutes, and quads similarly to the stomach muscle agencies or middle.

nine. Side Lunge- This stretch is fantastic for the hips and groin. Place your proper hand on right knee and slowly lunge to the proper. Move forward and repeat at the left component.

10. Shoulder Stretch- Pull your proper arm inside the course of your chest (proper bicep to chest). Apply moderate stress to higher arm. Feel the stretch to your shoulder. Repeat at the left element.

11. Triceps' Stretch- Reach decrease back and area proper palm in among shoulder blades. Apply mild strain with left hand on proper elbow. Move forward and repeat on the left issue.

12. Arm Circles- There is each other high-quality shoulder stretch to prepare your better frame for such sports activities sports as swimming, baseball or softball. Start off through circling right arm in clockwise movement on the issue of body. Repeat motion at the left element. Continue shifting forward alternating with clockwise and counter clockwise actions. It is likewise a good concept to transport from huge circles to smaller circles again to huge circles.

Static Stretching

While dynamic stretching is the notable manner to start your exercise, static stretching is the popular technique to cease your exercising. Static stretching facilitates get rid of the lactic acid constructing up that has came about in some unspecified time in the future of rigorous workout. It additionally allows to alleviate strain at the muscle mass similarly to growth your fashion of movement. Injury prevention is some different key purpose to spend a while on static stretching.

Static stretching has received a awful rap during the last decade or . Critics maintain that it takes too prolonged to finish. Many instances static stretching is not completed well, and for maximum humans it consequences in a completely unproductive flexibility session. With the exception of tune and bypass-united states teams, it has actually disappeared from many group and individual interest practices. The fact is that static stretching need to although be a very important thing in all mission and exercising sports. When you remain focused and anti-social, a static stretching regular may be completed in as low as twenty minutes time. There is no higher manner to forestall your exercising or exercising. As an added bonus static stretching can assist increase your stride period and make you a quicker runner. Let's take a look at the static stretching regular. Static Stretching Routine

The large difference among static and dynamic stretching workout workouts isn't always simplest on the entire time spent stretching, however moreover at the duration of time spent keeping the elongation of the muscle. A focused static stretch is completed over a minimum thirty second term and achieved for at least gadgets. You in no way need to bop and also you never want to gather a factor of pain. It may also moreover feel uncomfortable, however it ought to never be painful. The stretch is maintained for the whole thirty-2d time period, after which ought to be cushty earlier than performing the subsequent set. Here are a few essential static stretching bodily video video games. Again, you can pick out out and pick out those that preserve the maximum fee for you. Ideally the ones which are right now related to the interest you are involved in. Here are the static sports activities:

1. Hamstring Stretch- This is possibly one of the maximum critical stretches because it gives especially along side your middle and again. Sit on the floor together with your right leg prolonged out inside the front of you. Place the heel of the left foot at the facet of your right knee. Now, obtain your chest over your proper knee; concurrently gain every fingers over your right foot. Repeat collectively with your left leg. Make positive the stretch is extremely good felt within the hamstring (the returned of your leg).

2. Groin Stretch- Sit collectively along with your heels together inside the the front of you. Push down gently on your knees collectively with your elbows as you slowly

pull your ft to your groin. Your chest have to flow into out over your toes.

3.   Piriformis/Glutes Stretch- Wrap your proper leg round your left thigh on the same time as in a seated position. Now, slowly pull your knee toward your nose till you experience a stretch in your butt. Switch legs.

4.   Iliotibial Band Stretch- Lying for your yet again region your proper knee in a ninety diploma mindset above your face. Put your left knee on pinnacle of your right ankle. Now capture behind your left knee, and slowly pull your leg in the course of your face. The stretch must be felt inside the outside of your right hip, and deep inner your right glute. Now switch legs.

5.   Quadriceps Stretch- Standing tall, keep close your right ankle and raise your knee high within the lower lower back of your body. Now transfer legs. It is extraordinarily critical to experience this stretch to your quad or the front of your leg, and no longer on your knee. If you war with balance you can place

your opposite hand on a partner's shoulder or a wall to maintain balance.

6.   Calf Stretch- Lunge in advance along side your left knee at the identical time as status. Stay tall along with your better frame, and ensure your chest is ahead. Now, on the facet of your proper leg right now at the back of you, try to location your left heel on the ground. Hold the stretch after which transfer legs. This stretch may also be finished via leaning ahead in the course of a wall while you are reputation tall. Simply collect once more with every leg as you lean forward and try to press every heel to the ground. Stretch need to be felt inside the calf, the muscle located within the returned of your lower leg.

7.   Abdominals/ Lower Back- Lie in your stomach and slowly push your higher frame off the floor as your decrease body keeps touch with the ground. Keep your eyes and head beforehand as your palms stay right now.

eight. Groin/ Adductor Stretch- Stand tall together together with your ft approximately 3-five toes aside. Lean to the proper setting your right hand on right knee, and your left hand on left hip. Repeat on the other side.

nine. Hip/Trunk Twist- Stand tall with eyes up at the identical time as slowly turning on your right, on the identical time keep your feet dealing with forward. Repeat this on the left facet. Feet need to be approximately 2-3 feet aside.

10. Triceps Stretch- Reach decrease lower back with proper palm in amongst shoulder blades. Apply gentle, steady pressure along side your left hand on proper elbow. Repeat this at the opportunity issue.

eleven. Shoulder Stretch- Pull the proper arm across your body (bicep towards chest). Apply moderate, everyday pressure with left hand on right elbow. Repeat on the alternative element.

12. Arm Circles- Lift hands as masses as shoulder degree on each sides of your body. Begin the exercising with small clockwise circles progressively running your way up to massive circles. Repeat those actions in a counter clockwise motion.

thirteen. Chest/Shoulder/ Biceps Stretch-Clasp fingertips in the back of your decrease returned. Slowly growth clasped palms inside the course of the sky. Stay tall collectively collectively along with your eyes looking ahead.

14. Wrist and Hands Stretch- This stretch is incredible for any hobby that requires the usage of arms and decrease arms. Grab your right fingertips with the left hand and pull hands once more slowly. Repeat with the left arm. Stretching ought to be felt in wrist and arms. Finish with wrist rolls clockwise and counter clockwise.